THE FUNDAMENTALS OF NUTRITION AND HEALTH

ALICIA SINCLAIR
LANA ZINGER

KE KENDALL/HUNT PUBLISHING COMPANY
4050 Westmark Drive   Dubuque, Iowa 52002

Printed in the United States of America
10 9 8 7 6 5

TABLE OF CONTENTS

INTRODUCTION TO NUTRITION

Nutrition is a much talked about subject. Everyday, you hear nutrition messages from the media and sort through information from advertisers who want you to buy their products. Some products are healthy, but others may be lacking in nutrients. Sometimes it is difficult to sort it all out. Although many of us are aware that a healthy diet can prevent disease, not enough of us know about the healing powers of food. Proper nutrition helps regulate behavior, increase energy, and boost mood. With the right vitamins, minerals, essential fatty acids, and amino acids, people can begin to fight all sorts of conditions from cancer to heart disease. Nutrition awareness can help people make healthy food choices.

Maintaining Proper Nutrition Can:
- Give you stamina and energy for life
- Help you maintain an ideal body weight
- Boost your immune system
- Improve sports performance
- Delay the effects of aging
- Keep you active and fit into old age
- Help beat fatigue
- Protect teeth and keep gums healthy
- Enhance your ability to concentrate
- Alter mood
- Ward off serious illnesses like heart disease, certain cancers, diabetes type 2, and gallbladder disease

What is your definition of nutrition?

_____

_____

_____

_____

_____

_____

Ask someone what comes to mind when they hear the word *nutrition,* and most people respond: "diets," "vitamins," "healthy foods." Few people realize that nutrition is actually a science because nutrition as a discipline is fairly new. Nutrition has only been studied for roughly a century. People are bombarded with so many weight loss messages that few recognize it as a true science. In fact, **nutrition** is:

A new science that borrows from other sciences (i.e., chemistry, anatomy and physiology, biochemistry, and microbiology) that looks at the relationship between the foods we eat and our health.

To put a timeframe into perspective, the 100 years since 1890 were a large period of growth of the science of nutrition. Several key events took place during 1907 to 1919:

- E.V. McCollum (Sommer, 1989) and Adelle Davis (Harper, 1991) discovered fat-soluble vitamin A in butter and discovered water-soluble vitamin B in wheat germ.
- Axel Holst and Theodor Frolich were pioneers in the combat of scurvy by discovering an antiscorbutic substances (vitamin C) in fresh vegetables (Norum & Gray, 2002).
- By experimenting with fish oils, Edward Mellanby discovered a substance (vitamin D) to prevent rickets (Mellanby & Cantag, 1919).

By 1920, the science of nutrition was beginning to add reliable information about relationships between diet and health. These pivotal "discoveries" set the stage for the next several decades of nutrient research.

Why Good Nutrition Is Important

- **People are dying from unhealthy eating and inactivity.** According to the U.S. Department of Health and Human Services, unhealthy eating and inactivity cause **310,000 to 580,000 deaths every year,** which is similar to the number of deaths caused by tobacco and 13 times more than are caused by guns.
- **Quality of life is reduced.** Unhealthy eating and physical inactivity are major contributors to reduced quality of life and disabilities.
- **Almost two-thirds (61%) of American adults are overweight or obese.** Obesity rates in children have doubled in the last two decades, prompting concern about the rates of diet- and inactivity-related diseases that will occur as obese children age.
- **Diet and inactivity-related diseases are expensive.** Better nutrition could reduce the cost of heart disease, cancer, stroke, and diabetes by **$71 billion** each year.

Good Nutrition Provides Energy

The foods that you eat provide the energy that your body needs to function. Just like you need to put fuel in your car or recharge your cell phone battery, your body needs to be fed energy-providing foods every day. The main form of energy for your body is carbohydrates.

Good Nutrition Provides Muscles

Protein in the foods you that eat is broken down into individual amino acids. Your body uses the amino acids to build and repair the various parts of your body. Your muscles contain lots of protein, and you must replenish that protein through your diet. Your body also needs protein for components of your immune system, hormones, nervous system, and organs.

Your body also needs fats to be healthy. Membranes that contain fats surround all the cells of your body. Your brain has fatty acids, and fats are also needed to signal hormones.

Good Nutrition Provides Vitamins, Minerals and Other Helpers

Vitamins and minerals that you get from your diet are just as important as carbohydrates, protein, and fats; however, you only need vitamins and minerals in small amounts. Vitamins and minerals usually function as coenzymes, which mean they help chemical reactions in the body happen a lot faster. For example, many of the B complex vitamins help your body burn carbohydrates for energy. Vitamin A is needed for vision, zinc is involved in many metabolic processes, and vitamin C helps keep connective tissue strong and your immune system functioning.

Phytochemicals are found in the colorful parts of fruits and vegetables. Although they are not required for body functioning, they may have a very powerful impact on your health. For example, quercetin, which is found in red apples functions like an antihistamine and as an anti-inflammatory effect. Resveratrol, which is found in grape skins and seeds, is a powerful antioxidant. Antioxidants help protect your body from free radical damage that comes from the sun, pollution, smoke, and poor dietary choices. They are found in the phytochemicals of fruits and vegetables, as well as some vitamins and amino acids.

HOW POWERFUL IS A NUTRITIOUS DIET IN PREVENTING DISEASE?

So, is there a relationship between the foods that we eat and our health? You bet! Many disease states are associated with the foods that we eat. The choices that we make on a daily basis can, over time, wreak havoc on our health and have dire consequences. Malnutrition occurs if our bodies fail to get all the nutrients they need. If a person suffers from malnutrition he or she may be more likely to contract diseases. Malnutrition can affect the functions of their body such as brain, eyesight, organs, height, weight, as well as the formation of body parts if the child is still in its mother's womb. In the developing world, the biggest concerns often lie with the lack of vitamins and minerals, as well as the access to clean drinking water. According to the United Nations Children's Fund (UNICEF), almost one third of children in developing countries are malnourished. In addition to the shortage of food, disease also causes malnutrition. Diseases such as diarrhea cause the body to lose essential nutrients, by flushing them out of the body. Nutrients can take a long time to replace and may affect a child's growth and development.

In the United States, malnutrition is less of a problem as over nutrition and lifestyle diseases associated with eating too much or eating the wrong types of food. Lifestyle choices or modifiable behaviors are major causes of mortality in the United States. A lifestyle choice, or modifiable behavior is something that a person has some control over whether or not he or she will do that behavior.

In the United States, more than one third of all deaths can be attributed to a limited number of largely preventable behaviors and exposures including smoking, poor diet, physical inactivity and alcohol consumption. Like tobacco, obesity and inactivity increase the risks for the top three killers: heart disease, cancer, and cerebrovascular ailments including strokes. Obesity and inactivity also strongly increase the risk of diabetes, the sixth leading cause of death.

By the time they reach early adulthood, a large proportion of American youth have begun the poor practices contributing to three leading causes of preventable death in the United States: smoking, physical inactivity, and alcohol abuse. This finding is according to an analysis of the most comprehensive survey of adolescent health behavior undertaken to date by the National Institutes of Health (NIH). The analysis also found that significant health disparities exist between racial groups, and that Americans are less likely to have access to health care when they reach adulthood than they did during the teenage years.

Fast food and larger portions of it are taking a toll in the United States, where the surgeon general says 60 percent of adults are overweight or obese, as are nearly 13 percent of children. The prevalence of excess weight and obesity has nearly doubled among children and adolescents since 1980, and is increasing in both sexes and among all adults. The trends are already associated with major increases in the prevalence of conditions such as asthma and type 2 diabetes mellitus in children.

Changing modifiable behaviors can increase a person's life expectancy or longevity and prevent early deaths (McGinnis & Foege, 1993).

The following diseases are associated with poor diet:

- Hypertension
- Coronary artery disease
- Type II diabetes
- Osteoporosis
- Certain types of cancer, such as breast and colon cancer
- Obesity
- Elevated blood lipid levels

Leading Causes of Death

Rank*	Causes of death in 2004
	All causes
1.	Diseases of heart
2.	Malignant neoplasms (cancer)
3.	Cerebrovascular diseases
4.	Chronic lower respiratory diseases
5.	Unintentional injuries
6.	Diabetes mellitus
7.	Alzheimer's disease
8.	Influenza and pneumonia
9.	Nephritis, nephrotic syndrome, and nephrosis
10.	Septicemia

*Source: U.S. National Center for Health Statistics, *Health, United States, 2007.*

NUTRIENTS

The discipline of nutrition looks at the relationship between the foods we eat and one's health. Specifically, nutrition is concerned with *nutrients*. **Nutrients** are:

Substances found in food that help promote the growth and maintenance of the body.

When thinking about "growth and maintenance" of the body, many people think, "But, I'm *done* growing!" And, for people 18 years and older, this is true in its literal sense. However, the human body is growing and maintaining on a daily basis. The foods that we eat, which are made up of nutrients, help the body perform vital functions on a cellular level. For example, hair, skin, and nails are all made up of the nutrients in the foods we eat. Nutrients (such as protein) also help make certain hormones, like insulin, which helps regulate our blood sugar levels. We literally become the nutrients that we eat! If you eat a lot of junk food, your body's tissues are unhealthy. If you eat a lot of good-for-you foods, your body's tissues are healthy.

Six essential nutrients exist. "Essential" here means that the body cannot make on its own. In other words, the only way for us to get nutrients is by eating them. Each nutrient will be discussed in more detail in later chapters.

1. *Carbohydrate*

   Carbohydrates are the body's preferred fuel source and are found in plant-based foods like pasta, bread, rice, and fruits and vegetables.

2. *Lipid*

   Lipid is the chemical name for a family of fatty substances. In other words, lipids are fats and oils. Examples include different plant oils like olive or canola. Butter and lard are also examples of a lipid.

3. *Protein*

   Protein helps build and repair the body. Foods rich in protein include beef, poultry, fish, dairy, eggs and some plant foods like beans and nuts.

4. *Vitamins*

   Vitamins are substances the body needs in small amounts. Vitamins, along with minerals, act like spark plugs on a car's engine. Vitamins help the body perform vital tasks and prevent serious illness. Examples include vitamins A, D, E, K, and C; folate; niacin; thiamin; and riboflavin.

5. *Minerals*

   Minerals are substances the body needs in small amounts. Some examples include calcium, fluoride, and iodine.

6. *Water*

   Water is absolutely vital to all bodily functions. Water can be consumed in its pure form or through other beverages like milk, juice, or tea.

The first three nutrients—*carbohydrate, lipid,* and *protein*—are a little different than the last three (vitamins, minerals and water). They are often collectively referred to as "energy-yielding nutrients." Think of energy not as in "Rah, Rah! I'm so excited and energetic!" but instead think of **energy** as:

The capacity to do work.

What kind of "work" do you do each day? Take a moment and list all the activities that you do (for example, I walk to class). All of this work requires energy that allows you to move from point A to point B. This all happens because of the energy-yielding nutrients. Carbohydrates, lipid, and protein are considered energy yielding specifically because they contain calories and break them down to yield energy the body can use. For our purposes, you can think of a **calorie** as:

The measurement of a food's energy value.

On a more scientific level, a calorie is a measurement of heat. Specifically, food energy is measured in kilocalories (1,000 calories equal 1 kilocalorie) often abbreviated kcalories or kcal. A capitalized version is also sometimes used: Calories. One **kcalorie** is:

**The amount of heat necessary to raise the temperature of 1 kilogram (kg)
of water 1 degree Celsius** (Whitney & Rolfes, 1996).

The energy content of a particular food depends on how much of each of the energy-yielding nutrients it contains. Once completely broken down in the body, 1 gram (g) of carbohydrate yields about 4 kilocalories of energy; a gram of protein also yields 4 kcalories and 1 gram of lipid yields 9 calories! This is *more than* twice as many calories as a gram of carbohydrate or protein, respectively!

One other substance yields energy once when broken down in the body, yet it is not considered a nutrient because it does not help promote the growth and maintenance of the body (remember the definition of nutrient previously discussed): alcohol. One gram of alcohol yields 7 kilocalories. Quite a lot!

Remember the following list:

1 gram of carbohydrate = 4 kilocalories

1 gram of protein = 4 kilocalories

1 gram of lipid = 9 kilocalories

1 gram of alcohol = 7 kilocalories

Let's say you have a Mystery Candy Bar. It contains 22 grams of carbohydrate, 3 grams of protein, and 12 grams of lipid. How many total kilocalories does it contain?

22g × 4 = 88

3g × 4 = 12

12g × 9 = 108

TOTAL = 208 kcals

Let's try another one:

A Mystery Bag of Chips contains 31 grams of carbohydrate, 4 grams of protein and 10 grams of lipid. How many total kilocalories does it contain?

31g × ??

4g × ??

10g × ??

TOTAL = ??

Many people have the misconception that vitamins and minerals are what give them energy. Have you ever felt tired or run down and been told, "Oh, you just need your vitamins." Nothing could be further from the truth. Vitamins and minerals do not yield energy in the body once broken down. Because of this, they cannot provide you with the capacity to do work. So we've just "busted" a myth: **vitamins and minerals do not provide or enhance energy!**

Another key point when learning about the six essential nutrients is to recognize that protein and carbohydrate contain the same kilocalories per gram. This is surprising to people especially given the anti-carbohydrate craze currently popular in the United States. Keep in mind that one gram of lipid contains more than twice as many kilocalories as a gram each of carbohydrate and protein.

What does this mean for weight loss and/or weight gain? More will be discussed in later chapters, but for now, remember the following: **If you consume more food calories than your body requires, those calories will be stored as fat; if you consume fewer calories than your body requires, your body will draw on stored fat reserves and you will lose weight.**

Does this mean a person can gain weight by eating apples? Yes! Although it is much harder to gain weight eating apples than, say, a candy bar, if you consume more food calories than your body needs, no matter where it comes from, you store it as body fat.

How Many Calories Do *You* Need?

Each person has an allotted caloric value. In other words, each of us needs a certain amount of food in a given 24-hour time period. This amount is *highly variable* from person to person. Still, there are three main factors that help determine the number of food calories that should be eaten every day. Those factors are:

1. *Thermic Effect of Food*

   The thermic effect of food in its most simple definition is the amount of calories burned through the acts of digestion and absorption. Experts agree that this can account for roughly 5 percent to 10 percent of energy requirements. In other words, if you need 2,000 calories to maintain your current weight, you can assume that roughly 100 to 200 of those calories will be expended, thanks to the thermic effect of food.

2. *Physical Activity*

   Think about it: who burns more calories each day? Someone who has a desk job or someone whose job requires a lot of footwork like a nurse or a construction worker? Simply put, the more physically active you are, the more food you are able to consume and still maintain your weight.

   As we get older, we are less likely to be as active as we once were during our youth. That pick-up game of basketball or aerobics class after work fall to the way side when other adult responsibilities, like caring for children and paying household bills, take hold. The problem, however, is that people continue to eat the same amount of food as they did when they were more active. Was there any sort of change in the person's metabolic rate? Not really. The change is in the fact that the person no longer exercises the way he or she did previously. As a result, there is a decrease in muscle mass, which means the person is burning fewer calories at rest. All of these factors can contribute to age-related weight gain.

3. *Basal Metabolic Rate*

   Basal metabolic rate is the amount of calories that your body requires in a state of rest. Let's say you are in a car accident tomorrow and you are in the hospital lying in a coma. Do you still need to eat? Of course! Do you need as many food calories as you did before you were lying in a coma? No.

   What do you need the calories for if you are just lying there? All of your body's involuntary activities, like your kidneys filtering, heart pumping, and intestines digesting, require "fuel" to take place.

   Several factors affect your body's basal metabolic rate, and these factors are what make each of us different.

   - *Height*

   In general, the taller a person is, the higher their basal metabolic rate. Imagine if you owned a small studio apartment and a four floor townhouse. Which property would require more fuel to heat? The townhouse would because taller structures simply have more surface area and as a result require a lot of fuel.

- *Body Temperature*

  Have you ever heard the old wives' tale, "Feed a fever, starve a cold"? A person with a fever has a slightly increased basal metabolic rate. Normal body temperature is 98.6 degrees Fahrenheit. For every one degree above normal body temperature rises, basal metabolic rate increases roughly 7 percent.

- *Pregnancy & Lactation*

  Basal metabolic rate rises during pregnancy. In fact, after the first trimester of pregnancy, a woman requires an additional 300 kilocalories per day. Similarly, breastfeeding burns roughly an additional 500 kilocalories per day.

- *Growth*

  If Donald Trump builds a new skyscraper, what are some of the raw materials he would need to do so? Nails, cement, metal, screws, plaster board, etc. If you "build" a child, what are some of the raw materials necessary? FOOD! When a child is essentially growing from a "single story house" to a "skyscraper," the basal metabolic rate will rise to accommodate this.

- *Physical Activity*

  Through physical activity, especially strength training, basal metabolic rate rises. This factor is especially important because it is the one over which we truly have control. If you wish to increase your basal metabolic rate, start lifting weights and doing some cardiovascular activity.

Now that we know a bit more about nutrients, calories, and basal metabolic rate, let's take a look at some factors that affect our food selection on a regular basis.

Describe how you make food choices on a daily basis? Do you feel that you are in control of your food selection? Explain.

_____

_____

_____

_____

_____

_____

_____

_____

_____

_____

_____

_____

WHY DO WE EAT THE FOODS WE DO?

Every day, people make food choices, often without giving it much thought. Do you ever think about why you eat? The easy answers are because you are hungry, tired and your stomach is rumbling. Sometimes you might eat because you are bored, sad or happy; because it's lunchtime; or because that donut looks so good. Yet, if you dig a little deeper, most people have reasons behind their food selections whether they realize them or not.

Taste

Many people choose foods on taste alone. If it tastes good, eat it! Taste is largely determined by our genetics (Drayna, 2005). In other words, you've inherited a taste predisposition from your parents.

Children under 6 years old have abundant amounts of highly sensitive taste buds, which helps explain why they're often picky eaters. It is crucial that parents keep offering children, especially toddlers, a new food over and over again. Experts in pediatric nutrition point out that it may take up to 15 to 20 times for some children to be exposed to a food before they decide they like it.

When it comes to introducing new foods, the example set by you and by your child's peers can play a significant role. What kids see you eat becomes more acceptable to them. They are also more open to things they see other kids eating.

Cost

After taste, cost is a major factor behind food selection. The year 2008 has seen significant shifts in food costs. Sky-high food prices are being seen globally. In Pakistan, wheat is being stockpiled and its military is guarding flour mills. Indonesian consumers have taken to the streets to protest rising soy prices. Malaysia no longer lets people take sugar, flour, or cooking oil out of the country. North Dakota, the top U.S. wheat-producing state, may import from Canada due to tight supplies (Kirchoff & Waggoner, 2008)

Soaring demand along with rising oil prices have sent many commodity prices to their highest levels in history. Prices for some varieties of wheat are at an all-time high of more than $16 a bushel on the Minneapolis Grain Exchange. Corn, which has averaged about $2.50 per bushel in recent years, is above $5 in 2008.

According to the Bureau of Labor Statistics, in 2006, bread cost $1.05 per pound. In 2008, bread cost $1.28 per pound. Apples in 2006 cost 96 cents per pound. In 2008, they cost $1.16 per pound. In 2006, a dozen eggs cost $1.45. In 2008, they cost $2.18.

What does all of this mean for consumers? Unfortunately, as Americans face these rising foods costs, more and more people will turn to unhealthy, low-quality sources, like fast-food restaurants and vending machines (Frazao, 1999). They may also skip meals altogether or forgo staples such as bread and dairy.

One way to combat soaring food costs is to shop at local green markets, a trend that has increased in the past decade. Green markets offer fresh, locally grown foods that tend to be cheaper than regular grocery stores because the food didn't have to be shipped long distances.

Convenience and Availability

In addition to financial feasibility, people eat foods that are accessible, quick, and easy to prepare. In 2006, Americans reported eating out approximately five times a week. Fast-food restaurants were the most popular eating establishments for breakfast and lunch, and fast-food and casual dining were the two most popular places for dinner. Ease, convenience, and cost were among the top reasons respondents ordered value/combo meals at fast-food restaurants (*Science Daily*, 2007). Unfortunately, all of this eating out can lead to dire health consequences.

Emotional Comfort

Americans are notorious for their love of food. We eat when we are happy, sad, angry, bored, lonely, anxious, and depressed. The one time we *should* eat is when we are truly hungry and we often don't. Hunger is the biological urge to eat, which is often felt below the neck. Appetite, on the other hand, is the psychological urge to eat, often "felt" above the neck. When people regularly consume food for comfort, it can lead to obesity and all of the health problems associated with overweight and obesity.

Culture/Family Background

Among the strongest factors behind food selection is a person's ethnic and cultural heritage. Simply put, people eat the foods they grew up eating.

Health and Body Weight

With more than 60 percent of adult Americans overweight or obese, it is no surprise that body weight is a factor behind a person's food selection. It's vital, however, that the person has a firm grasp on basic nutritional principles to help make healthy food choices.

WHAT DOES A NUTRITIOUS DIET LOOK LIKE?

Americans are always looking for a "quick fix" or the latest diet to follow or pill to take to solve their weight woes. In fact, a nutritious diet in its most simple form is easy to follow and has four basic characteristics. They are:

1. *Adequate*

   Adequate is a word that does not often come to mind, but in fact, most Americans are malnourished. They eat a lot, but a lot of the *wrong* foods. An adequate diet is one that ensures enough of the "good stuff" like fiber, protein, fruits, vegetables, and whole grains. An adequate diet limits, or avoids altogether, foods that are highly processed or refined.

2. *Balanced*

   Think back to when you learned about the different food groups. A balanced diet is one that incorporates all five food groups:

   - Fruits
   - Vegetables, including legumes and nuts
   - Whole grains
   - Low-fat dairy
   - Lean meats, poultry, and seafood

     Diets that propose eliminating an entire food group are not balanced and, unless there is a medical reason for doing so, can result in poor health.

3. *Varied*

   The term varied is sometimes confused with balanced, but they are different concepts as they relate to a person's diet. A varied diet includes a wide selection of foods. For example, say you bring a red delicious apple with you to lunch everyday. One way to vary this would be to bring a golden delicious apple one day, and the next day bring a granny smith apple, and the next day try switching to a new fruit altogether! Do not be afraid to experiment with eating new foods. The point is that by eating a varied diet, you ensure that you are consuming many different nutrients.

4. *Moderate*

   Moderate is probably the most important characteristic of all. Look at the diets of other countries. The French, for example, eat a wide selection of foods such as fruits, vegetables, and whole grains, but they also consume butter, chocolate, and cheese. Then why are they so slim compared to Americans? Moderation is the answer. A moderate diet is one that avoids excess. In other words, you may include your favorite "junk" foods in your daily diet. In fact, doing so means you are less likely to binge on these foods. The key, however, is to do so in moderation. Have one or two cookies, not the whole sleeve. Have a scoop of ice cream, not the whole pint. Have a slice or two of pizza, not the whole pie. One way to practice this is by listening to your body's cues. It will tell you when it is hungry. It will also tell you when it is satisfied. Once you get used to this—and it may take some time, especially if you are a member of the "clean your plate club"—your weight will naturally fall within its normal range.

This is really all healthy eating boils down to—an adequate, balanced, varied and moderate diet. If you were to follow these principles, along with some moderate exercise, your weight should fall in a normal range for your height and genetics. The next time you, a friend, or a family member want to jump on the latest diet craze, remember these four characteristics, which will sustain you for life.

Because we are bombarded with nutrition news in newspapers, magazines, television, online, or just by talking with friends, it's more important than ever that we can believe in and safely use nutrition news we hear about. Unfortunately, the "expert" most people turn to for nutrition advice (i.e., a doctor) may not be the best person to help guide you. Only about one-fourth of all medical schools in the United States require students to take even one nutrition course (Shils, 1994). Today this is changing slowly, but surely. Still, physicians are burdened with many responsibilities and few will take the time, or truly have the expertise, to develop detailed diet plans for their patients. Instead, physicians often refer patients to registered dieticians, who are the appropriate qualified nutrition experts.

What Is a Registered Dietitian?

A registered dietician has the educational background necessary to deliver nutrition education and advice. To become a registered dietitian, a person must follow a rigorous bachelor's degree program with an emphasis in the sciences and clinical nutrition courses. During the final year of the bachelor's training, the student will follow a two-semester internship at various sites: clinical, community, and food service. Once these requirements have been met, the student must pass a national certification exam, indicating competency in core areas of dietetics.

By educating people about the connection between food and health, nutritionists and dietitians promote good eating habits to help prevent disease and to treat preexisting conditions.

Responsibilities of a Clinical Dietician
(Adapted by Whitney & Rolfes, 1996)

- Assesses clients' nutrition status.
- Determines clients' nutrient requirements.
- Monitors clients' nutrient intakes.
- Develops, implements, and evaluates clients' nutrition care plans.
- Counsels clients to cope with unique diet plans.
- Teaches clients and their families about nutrition and diet plans.
- Provides training for other dietitians, nurses, interns, and dietetics students.
- Serves as a liaison between clients and the food service department.
- Communicates with physicians, nurses, pharmacists, and other health care professionals about clients' progress, needs, and treatments.
- Participates in professional activities to enhance knowledge and skill.

ASSIGNMENT #1

Name: _____

Date: _____

1. Describe your current eating habits.

_____

_____

_____

_____

_____

_____

_____

_____

_____

_____

2. What are your nutrition goals? Are you satisfied with your eating habits?

_____

_____

_____

_____

_____

_____

_____

_____

_____

_____

3. How do you rate your eating habits based on the dietary guidelines?

_____

_____

_____

_____

_____

_____

_____

_____

4. Based on the dietary guidelines, choose one thing you would like to change in your current diet, and describe why it's important to make the change.

_____

_____

_____

_____

_____

_____

_____

_____

_____

_____

_____

_____

_____

_____

_____

_____

_____

_____

_____

_____

_____

_____

RESOURCES

Bureau of Labor Statistics: http://www.bls.gov/ Page 13, 3rd paragraph.

Drayna, D. (2005). *Human Taste Genetics.* Vol. 6: 217–235.

Frazao, E. High Costs of Poor Eating Patterns in the United States. In *America's Eating Habits: Changes and Consequences.* Economic Research Service, U.S. Department of Agriculture. Washington, DC: USDA, 1999. Agriculture Information Bulletin No. 750, pp. 5–32.

Harper, A. E. (1991). *American Journal of Clinical Nutrition;* 53: 413–20.

Norum, K. R., Gray, H. J. (2002). Axel Holst and Theodor Frolich—Pioneers in the combat of scurvy. *Tidsskr Nor Laegeforen:* June 30; 122(17); 1686–7.

Kirchhoff, S., Waggoner, J. (2008). *USA Today:* February 11, 2008.

McGinnis, J. M., Foege, W. H. (1993). Actual Causes of Death in the United States. *Journal of the American Medical Association* Vol. 270, no. 18: 2207–2212.

Mellanby, E. & Cantag, M. D. (1919). Experimental investigation on rickets. *Lancet* 196: 407–412.

Science Daily: Price and taste trump nutrition when Americans eat out. October 23, 2007.

Shils, M. E. (1994). Nutrition education in medical schools—the prospect before us. *American Journal of Clinical Nutrition;* Oct; 60(4):631–8.

Sommer, A. (1989). New Imperatives for an Old Vitamin. *Journal of Nutrition:* Vol. 119 No. 1: 96–100.

United Nations Children's Fund (UNICEF). http://www.unicef.org/index.php.

United States National Center for Health Statistics (2007), *Health,* United States.

Whitney, E. N., Rolfes, S. R. (1996). Understanding Nutrition 7th Edition. West Publishing Company.

THE NEW DIETARY GUIDELINES: PRACTICAL ADVICE FOR HEALTHIER LIVING

HISTORY OF USDA'S FOOD GUIDANCE

The U.S. Department of Agriculture (USDA) has had a long history with food guidance dating back into the early twentieth century. Looking back over this history, many different food guides have been used. All of these food guides preceded the introduction of the original food guide pyramid in 1992.

> 1916: Food for Young Children
>
> 1940s: National Food Guide (commonly called "The Basic Seven")
>
> 1950s–1960s: Food for Fitness—A Daily Food Guide (commonly called "The Basic Four")
>
> 1970s: Hassle-Free Guide to a Better Diet
>
> 1992: Food Guide Pyramid
>
> 2005: MyPyramid

Before vitamins and minerals were even discovered, the USDA published its first dietary recommendations to the nation in 1894. In 1916, the first food guide, called Food for Young Children was published. Caroline Hunt, a nutritionist and the author, divided food into five groups: milk/meat, cereals, vegetables/fruits, fats/fatty foods, and sugars/sugary foods. Prompted by President Franklin Roosevelt, a National Nutrition Conference was called to action in 1941. For the first time, the USDA came up with Recommended Dietary Allowances (RDA's) for Americans to follow. In 1943, the USDA announced the "Basic Seven," which was a special modification of the nutritional guidelines to help people deal with the shortage of food supplies during the war.

Because of the complexity of the Basic Seven, the Basic Four was introduced and was used for the next 20 years. Milk, meats, fruits and vegetables, and grain products were the categories from which to eat foods. With chronic diseases like stroke and heart disease on the rise, the USDA needed to address the roles of unhealthy foods. During the late 1970s, the USDA added a fifth category to the Basic Four: fats, sweets, and alcoholic beverages, for people to consume in moderation.

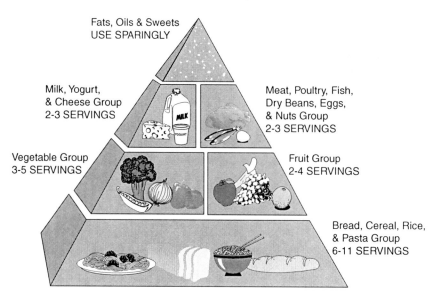

The Food Guide Pyramid

Fats, Oils & Sweets
USE SPARINGLY

Milk, Yogurt,
& Cheese Group
2-3 SERVINGS

Meat, Poultry, Fish,
Dry Beans, Eggs,
& Nuts Group
2-3 SERVINGS

Vegetable Group
3-5 SERVINGS

Fruit Group
2-4 SERVINGS

Bread, Cereal, Rice,
& Pasta Group
6-11 SERVINGS

Source: http://www.nal.usda.gov/fnic/Fpyr/pmap.htm

Although a "Pattern for Daily Food Choices," the USDA's food guide, had been published annually since the 1980's, many people were still not aware that it existed. Beginning in 1988, the USDA created a graphic to represent the food groups. The USDA needed to convey the three main ideas: variety, proportionality and moderation. The Food Guide Pyramid was finally released in 1992. Both the graphics and text conveyed variety and proportionality with pictures of foods and the size of the food group. In 1994, the Nutrition Labeling and Education Act required that every food in the grocery store have a nutritional label.

The Food Guide Pyramid was published in 1992 to replace the earlier food groups' classification system. Since that time, there has been an epidemic increase in type 2 diabetes which is now even afflicting a large and rapidly increasing number of children. The Food Guide Pyramid is an outline of what to eat each day based on the Dietary Guidelines. It is not a rigid prescription but instead a general guide that lets you choose a healthful diet that's right for you. The Pyramid calls for eating a variety of foods to get the nutrients you need and, at the same time, the right amount of calories to maintain healthy weight.

FAULTS OF THE USDA'S PYRAMID

Since the pyramid was released by the U.S. Department of Agriculture in 1992, nutrition scientists have criticized the content and design and proposed numerous alternatives, including the Harvard's Healthy Eating Pyramid. According to many scientists, the food pyramid is not up-to-date with current nutritional research. Harvard scientist Dr. Willet believes six faults of the food pyramid are misleading American people. Source: Willet,W. (2005) *Eat, Drink and Be Healthy: The Harvard Medical School Guide to Healthy Eating.*

1. **All fats are bad.** Not true! Only certain fats are bad for you (saturated and trans fats), while others (monosaturated and polyunsaturated fats) provide many benefits to your heart. Some of these good fats are found in nuts, fish, olive oil and whole grains.

2. **All complex carbohydrates are good.** Not true! The food pyramid recommends six to eleven servings of carbohydrates a day, which is way too much. It also does not differentiate between the two kinds of carbohydrates, simple carbohydrates (sugars) and complex carbohydrates (starches). The majority of a person's carbohydrate intake should come from whole grains (complex carbs), which will make you feel fuller longer and also give you a lot of fiber. Stay away from refined carbohydrates, which are things like cookies, crackers, and chips. If you eat those, eat them in moderation.

3. **Protein is protein.** Not true! Protein should be a key component of your diet. But some sources of protein are better for you than others. For example, red meat (steaks) may have a good amount of protein, but they also are high in cholesterol and saturated fat, which is not good for your heart. Fish, chicken, turkey, and pork are lower in saturated fat and have just as much protein. Even beans and nuts are great sources of protein that people wouldn't necessarily know about.

4. **Dairy products are essential.** Not true! Dr. Willett says that despite all the commercials advertising protection against osteoporosis, there really is not a calcium emergency in America. Our country gets more calcium than any other country. In reality, he says, there are even studies that suggest that drinking and/or eating a lot of dairy sources can possibly increase a man's chance of getting prostate cancer or a woman's chance of getting ovarian cancer. You still need some calcium in your diet, however you don't have to get it from milk or yogurt. Spinach, tofu, orange juice, and broccoli have calcium and extra nutrients. A calcium supplement, which may be cheaper and lower in calories than dairy products, is another way to add calcium to a diet.

5. **Eat your potatoes.** Not true! Potatoes are starches, not vegetables! A baked potato increases blood sugar levels and insulin faster and to higher levels than an equal amount of calories from pure table sugar. French fries are even worse. If you must eat potatoes, eat them in moderation.

6. **No guidance on weight, exercise, alcohol, and vitamins.** Although the food pyramid suggests how to plan a healthy diet, it does not mention four other key parts of maintaining a healthy body: the importance of not gaining weight, the necessity of daily exercise, the potential health benefits of a daily alcoholic drink, and what you can gain by taking a daily multivitamin.

The Harvard School of Public Health created an alternative to the USDA's food pyramid called the Healthy Eating Pyramid. One of the most interesting changes in this pyramid is that plant oils are half of the near bottom part of the pyramid shared with grains. Harvard is stressing the importance of the right fats and the fact that fat calories make up about 30 percent of a healthy diet. The inclusion on exercise and maintaining a healthy weight are very important aspects of nutrition and are stressed in the Healthy Eating Pyramid by putting these as the base.

Tips for Using the Harvard's Healthy Eating Pyramid

1. **Start with exercise.** A healthy diet is built on a base of regular exercise, which keeps calories in balance and weight in check.

2. **Focus on food, not grams.** The Healthy Eating Pyramid does not address specific servings or grams of food, so neither should you. It is a simple, general guide to how you should eat when you eat.

3. **Go with plants.** Eating a plant-based diet is healthiest. Choose plenty of vegetables, fruits, whole grains, and healthy fats, like olive and canola oil.

4. **Cut way back on American staples.** Red meat, refined grains, potatoes, sugary drinks, and salty snacks are part of American culture, but they are also really unhealthy. Go for a plant-based diet rich in non-starchy vegetables, fruits, and whole grains. If you eat meat, fish and poultry are the best choices.

5. **Take a multivitamin, and maybe have a drink.** Taking a multivitamin can be a good nutrition insurance policy. Moderate drinking for many people can have real health benefits, but it is not for everyone. Moderate alcohol consumption is defined as two drinks or less per day for men and one drink or less per day for women. One drink equals one shot, one beer or 4 oz of wine. Those who don't drink shouldn't feel that they need to start.

BASIC PRINCIPLES OF ALL FOOD PYRAMIDS

With the variety of food pyramids available, you may wonder which one to follow. It may help to know that the basic principles of food pyramids are largely the same and generally emphasize the following:

- Eat more fruits, vegetables, and whole grains.
- Reduce intake of saturated fat, trans fat, and cholesterol.
- Limit sweets and salt.
- Drink alcoholic beverages in moderation, if at all.
- Control portion sizes and the total number of calories that you consume.
- Include physical activity in your daily routine.
- Food pyramids place foods in categories such as dairy products or meat and beans, to help guide your food choices. No single food provides all of the nutrients that your body needs, so eating a variety of foods within each group ensures that you get the necessary nutrients and other substances that promote good health.

THE DIETARY GUIDELINES FOR AMERICANS

The *Dietary Guidelines for Americans* has been published jointly every five years since 1980 by the Department of Health and Human Services (HHS) and the Department of Agriculture (USDA). The *Dietary Guidelines for Americans* provide research-based dietary advice designed to promote health and reduce risk for the major chronic conditions and diseases that affect people in the United States., including obesity, diabetes, cardiovascular disease, high blood pressure, cancer, and osteoporosis. The Dietary Guidelines are the cornerstone of federal nutrition policy and influence the numerous food and nutrition programs of the federal government. These include the Food Stamp Program; Special Supplemental Nutrition Program for Women, Infants, and Children (WIC); National School Lunch Program; and School Breakfast Program. The latest edition of the dietary guidelines was introduced in 2005.

Two-thirds of Americans are overweight or obese, and more than 50 percent of Americans do not get the recommended amount of physical activity. In 2005 guidelines emphasize physical activity and calorie control more than ever before.

The dietary guidelines describe a healthy diet as one that:

- Emphasizes fruits, vegetables, whole grains, and fat-free or low-fat milk and milk products;
- Includes lean meats, poultry, fish, beans, eggs, and nuts; and
- Is low in saturated fats, trans fats, cholesterol, salt (sodium), and added sugars.

MyPyramid.gov

MyPyramid replaces the Food Guide Pyramid introduced in 1992. MyPyramid is part of an overall food guidance system that emphasizes the need for a more individualized approach to improving diet and lifestyle. The new food guidance system utilizes interactive technology found on www.mypyramid.gov. The interactive activities make it easy for individuals to enter their age, gender and physical activity level to obtain a more personalized recommendation on their daily calorie level based on the 2005 *Dietary Guidelines for Americans*. The web site features MyPyramid Plan, MyPyramid Tracker, and Inside MyPyramid, as well as tips, resources, as well as a worksheet.

MyPyramid food plans are designed for the general public ages 2 and over; they are not therapeutic diets.

ANATOMY OF MYPYRAMID

One Size Does Not Fit All

MyPyramid offers personalized eating plans, interactive tools to help you plan and assess your food choices, and advice to help you:

- Make smart choices from every food group.
- Find your balance between food and physical activity.
- Get the most nutrition out of your calories.
- Stay within your daily calorie needs.

Activity

Activity is represented by the steps and the person climbing them, as a reminder of the importance of daily physical activity.

Moderation

Moderation is represented by the narrowing of each food group from bottom to top. The wider base stands for foods with little or no solid fats or added sugars. These should be selected more often. The narrower top area stands for foods containing more added sugars and solid fats. The more active you are, the more of these foods can fit into your diet.

Personalization

Personalization is shown by the person on the steps, the slogan, and the URL, or web address. Find the kinds of amounts of food to eat each day at MyPyramid.gov.

Proportionality

Proportionality is shown by the different widths of the food group bands. The widths suggest how much food a person should choose from each group. The widths are just a general guide, not exact proportions. Check the web site for how much is right for you.

Variety

Variety is symbolized by the six color bands representing the five food groups of the Pyramid and oils. This illustrates that foods from all groups are needed each day for good health.

Gradual Improvement

Gradual improvement is encouraged by the slogan. It suggests that individuals can benefit from taking small steps to improve their diet and lifestyle each day.

DISCRETIONARY CALORIES

(A new concept first described by the 2005 Dietary Guidelines Advisory Committee)

> **Discretionary calories = Total estimated energy requirement – Essential calories**

When all food choices are in "nutrient-dense forms" that is lean or low-fat, with no added sugars then nutrient needs can be met with fewer calories than the amount required for energy balance. The calories needed to meet nutrient needs are called "essential calories." By subtracting the essential calories from a person's total energy requirements, the number of calories available for discretionary food choices can be determined. This remaining balance of discretionary calories permits some choices of foods with higher levels of fat and some added sugars intake, or increased intake from any food group. These amounts of "extras" however are lower than most Americans now consume.

As energy requirements increase with increased physical activity, the amount of discretionary calories increases.

Weight Management

If you are significantly overweight, you have a greater risk of developing many diseases, including high blood pressure, type 2 diabetes, stroke, and some forms of cancer. For obese adults, even losing a few pounds or preventing further weight gain has health benefits. Reaching a healthier weight is a balancing act. The secret is learning how to balance your "energy in" and "energy out" over the long run. "Energy in" is the calories from the foods and beverages you have each day. "Energy out" is the calories that you burn for basic body functions and physical activity.

Energy In = Energy Out

Your weight will stay the same when the calories that you eat and drink equal the calories that you burn.

Energy In < Energy Out

You will lose weight when the calories that you eat and drink are less than the calories that you burn.

Energy In > Energy Out

You will gain weight when the calories that you eat and drink are greater than the calories that you burn.

Physical Activity

For health benefits, physical activity should be **moderate** or **vigorous** and add up to at least 30 minutes a day. Everyone should get a minimum of 30 to 60 minutes each day of moderate exercise brisk walking or bicycling, for example. Losing weight will require 60 to 90 minutes of more intense daily exercise.

Moderate Physical Activities Include:
- Walking briskly (about 3 ½ miles per hour)
- Hiking
- Gardening/yard work
- Dancing
- Golf (walking and carrying clubs)
- Bicycling (less than 10 miles per hour)
- Weight training (general light workout)

Vigorous Physical Activities Include:
- Running/jogging (5 miles per hour)
- Bicycling (more than 10 miles per hour)
- Swimming (freestyle laps)
- Aerobics
- Walking very fast (4 ½ miles per hour)
- Heavy yard work, such as chopping wood
- Weight lifting (vigorous effort)
- Competitive basketball

Food Groups to Encourage:
- Eat fruits and vegetables for a total of at least 4.5 cups (9 servings) each day
- Choose low-fat or fat-free milk, yogurt, and other dairy products
- Try to eat at least half of your grains as whole grain foods, or about 3 ounce-equivalents each day

What Counts as One Serving?

The amount of food that counts as one serving is listed in the following table.

Be sure to eat at least the lowest number of servings from the five major food groups listed. You need them for the vitamins, minerals, carbohydrates, and protein that they provide. Just try to pick the lowest fat choices from the food groups. No specific serving size is given for the fats, oils, and sweets group because the message is use sparingly.

Milk, Yogurt, and Cheese		
1 cup of milk or yogurt	1 ½ ounces of natural cheese	2 ounces of process cheese

Meat, Poultry, Fish, Dry Beans, Eggs, and Nuts	
2 to 3 ounces of cooked lean meat, poultry, or fish	½ cup of cooked dry beans, 1 egg, or 2 tablespoons of peanut butter count as 1 ounce of lean meat

Vegetable		
1 cup of raw leafy vegetables	½ cup of other vegetables, cooked or chopped raw	¾ cup of vegetable juice

Fruit		
1 medium apple, banana, orange	½ cup of chopped, cooked, or canned fruit	¾ cup of fruit juice

Bread, Cereal, Rice, and Pasta		
1 slice of bread	1 ounce of ready-to-eat cereal	½ cup of cooked cereal, rice, or pasta

Protein

- Go lean with protein.
- Consider dry beans and peas as an alternative to meat or poultry.
- Keep the overall amounts of foods eaten from this group within the amount needed each day. For example, people who need 2,000 calories per day need 5 ½ ounce-equivalents per day.

Strategies for Protein

- Select meat cuts that are low in fat and ground beef that is extra lean (at least 90% lean).
- Trim fat from meat and removing poultry skin before cooking or eating.
- Drain fat from ground meats after cooking.
- Use preparation methods that do not add fat, such as grilling, broiling, poaching, or roasting.
- Choose lean turkey, roast beef, or ham or low-fat luncheon meats for sandwiches instead of fatty luncheon meats such as bologna or salami.

Consume a sufficient amount of fruits and vegetables while staying within your energy needs. Fruits and vegetables have a strong boost. Nine servings of produce are recommended for the average 2,000-calorie diet, which translates to 2 cups of fruit and 2 ½ cups of vegetables each day. Within the recommended 2 cups of fruit a day, whole fruit whether fresh, canned, frozen or dried is recommended rather than fruit juice to obtain an adequate amount of fiber.

Within the recommended 2 ½ cups of vegetables a day and whether you choose fresh, canned, or frozen you should include a variety from the following five subgroups throughout the week: dark green vegetables (spinach, most greens), legumes (dry beans, chickpeas), starchy vegetables (corn, green peas), orange vegetables (carrots, sweet potatoes), and other vegetables (tomatoes, green beans).

Strategies for Meeting Fruit Recommendation

- Use fruit in salads, toppings, desserts, and/or snacks regularly.
- Use fruit as a topping on cereal, pancakes, and other foods rather than sugars, syrups, or other sweet toppings.
- Select fruits that are in season to increase variety.
- Use canned, frozen, and dried fruits as well as fresh fruits.
- Avoid fruit canned in syrup. Light or heavy syrup adds sugar to canned fruits. Fruits canned in juice or water are a better choice.

Strategies for Vegetables

- Include vegetables in lunch, dinner, and snacks.
- Prepare main dishes, side dishes, and salads that include vegetables.
- Add vegetables to mixed dishes such as soups, stews, casseroles, and stir-fries
- Add dark-green or orange vegetables to soups, stews, casseroles, and stir-fries.
- Use romaine, spinach, or other dark leafy greens as salad greens, and eat green salads often.
- Choose main dishes, side dishes, and salads that include cooked dry beans or peas.

Milk, Yogurt, and Cheese

Calcium builds strong bones to last a lifetime, so you need these foods in your diet. Choose fat-free or low-fat milk, yogurt, and cheese. If you choose milk or yogurt that is not fat-free, or cheese that is not low-fat, the fat in the product counts as part of the discretionary calorie allowance. If you choose sweetened milk products e.g., flavored milk, yogurt, drinkable yogurt, desserts, you must count the added sugars as part of the discretionary calorie allowance.

For those who are lactose intolerant, lactose-free and lower-lactose products are available. Also, enzyme preparations can be added to milk to lower the lactose content.

Fats

Less than 10 percent of calories should come from saturated fats, and fat should make up no more than 25 to 30 percent of total calories. No firm guideline was set for trans fats, only a recommendation to keep them "as low as possible." The best sources should come from mainly polyunsaturated and monounsaturated fats: fish, nuts, vegetable oils.

Types of Fats

Saturated

- Meat
- Egg yolk
- Butter
- Dairy
- Coconut
- Palm oil

Polyunsaturated

- Vegetable oils
- Fish (omega-3s)
- Walnuts
- Almonds

Monounsaturated

- Olive oil
- Peanut oil
- Avocados

Trans Fats

- Labeled as "partially hydrogenated"

Strategies for Using Fats

- Choose "healthy fats" such as olive oil and canola oil.
- Use canola margarine and cook with canola oil.
- Use olive oil salad dressings.
- Avoid "unhealthy fats" such as saturated and trans fat.
- Check nutrition labels and ingredient lists.
- Choose low-fat dairy products and lean meats.
- Eat at least two seafood meals each week.
- Include a source of omega-3 fats.

Carbohydrates

The health benefits of eating whole grains include lowering the risk of:

- Coronary heart disease
- Type 2 diabetes
- Colon cancer
- Obesity

What Is a Whole Grain?

- Foods made with the entire grain seed (kernel).
- FDA health claim: Whole grain food must contain 51 percent or more whole grain ingredients by weight per reference amount and be low in fat and cholesterol
- *Refined grains* have been milled i.e., the bran and germ are removed. This process also removes much of the B vitamins, iron, and dietary fiber. Some refined grains are enriched. This means certain B vitamins (thiamin, riboflavin, niacin, folic acid) and iron are added back after processing. Fiber is not added back to most enriched grains.

Finding Whole Grains When Shopping

Good Source	A half serving (8g) of whole grain
Excellent Source	A full serving (16g) of whole grain
100%/Excellent	A full serving (16g) and all grains are whole

Examples of Whole Grains

- Amaranth
- Barley
- Brown rice
- Buckwheat
- Bulgur
- Kamut
- Millet
- Oatmeal
- Popcorn
- Quinoa
- Sorghum
- Spelt
- Whole corn
- Whole-grain pasta
- Whole rye
- Whole wheat
- Whole-wheat couscous
- Wild rice

Strategies for Consuming Carbohydrates

- Choose fiber-rich fruits, vegetables, and whole grains often.
- Choose and prepare foods and beverages with little added sugars or caloric sweeteners.
- Reduce the incidence of dental caries by consuming sugar- and starch-containing foods and beverages less frequently.

- Eat three or more ounce-equivalents of whole grain products per day.
- Half your grains should come from whole grains.

Sodium and Potassium
- Choose and prepare foods with little salt.
- Consume less than 2,300 mg (1 tsp salt) of sodium each day.
- Check food labels for sodium. Foods with less than 140 mg sodium (5% DV) are low in salt.

Consume Potassium-Rich Foods, Such as Fruits and Vegetables
- Some vegetables that are rich in potassium include sweet potatoes, beet greens, white potatoes, white beans, tomato products, soybeans, lima beans, winter squash, spinach, lentils, kidney beans, and split peas.
- Some fruits that are rich in potassium include prune juice, bananas, cantaloupe, honeydew, prunes, dried peaches or apricots, orange juice, and plantains. Some fruit juices, such as orange and prune juice, are rich in potassium.

Strategies for Sodium
- Beware that processed meats and fresh chicken, turkey, and pork that have been enhanced with a salt-containing solution also have added sodium.
- Beware that frozen dinners, packaged mixes, cereals, cheese, breads, soups, salad dressings, pickles, ketchup, olives and sauces have added sodium.
- Beware that foods with less than 140 mg sodium per serving can be labeled as "low sodium foods."

Food Guide Pyramid for Kids Ages 4 to 13

Grains
- 4- to 8-year-olds need 4 to 5 ounce equivalents each day.
- 9- to 13-year-old girls need 5 ounce equivalents each day.
- 9- to 13-year-old boys need 6 ounce equivalents each day.

Vegetables
- 4- to 8-year-olds need 1 ½ cups of vegetables each day.
- 9- to 13-year-old girls need 2 cups of vegetables each day.
- 9- to 13-year-old boys need 2 ½ cups of vegetables each day.

Fruits
- 4- to 8-year-olds need 1– to 1 ½ cups of fruit each day.
- 9- to 13-year-olds need 1 ½ cups of fruit each day.

Milk and Other Calcium-Rich Foods
- 4- to 8-year-olds need 2 cups of milk (or another calcium-rich food) each day.
- 9- to 13-year-olds need 3 cups of milk (or another calcium-rich food) each day.

Meats, Beans, Fish, and Nuts
- 4- to 8-year-olds need 3 to 4 ounce equivalents each day.
- 9- to 13-year-olds need 5 ounce equivalents each day.

ASSIGNMENT #2

Name: _____

Date: _____

Go to www.mypyramid.gov and click on mypyramid plan and then mypyramid menu planner. Enter your age, gender, and activity level to get your own plan at an appropriate calorie level. The food plan will include specific daily amounts from each food group and a limit for discretionary calories. Print out a personalized poster of your plan, and a worksheet to help you track your progress.

1. Describe your results, and compare it to your current eating habits.

_____
_____
_____
_____
_____
_____
_____
_____
_____
_____
_____
_____
_____
_____
_____
_____
_____
_____
_____
_____
_____
_____
_____
_____
_____
_____
_____
_____

2. What are your short-term and long-term nutrition goals based on the dietary guidelines?

_____

_____

_____

_____

_____

_____

_____

_____

_____

_____

_____

3. Rate your experience using mypyramid.gov. Is it user-friendly? Have you heard of it in the past?

_____

_____

_____

_____

_____

_____

_____

_____

_____

_____

_____

4. If you were creating a food pyramid/plan for Americans to follow, what would you do differently?

_____

_____

_____

_____

_____

_____

_____

_____

_____

_____

RESOURCES

Buzby J. C., Hodan F. W. and Vocke G. (2006). Possible Implications for U.S. Agriculture from Adoption of Select Dietary Guidelines. Economic Research Report No. ERR-31. Available at: http://www.ers.usda.gov/Publications/ERR31/.

Davis, C., Saltos, E. Dietary Recommendations and How They Have Changed Over Time. Available at: http://www.ers.usda.gov/publications/aib750/aib750b.pdf.

Family Health Administration: http://www.fha.state.md.us/ocd/cardio/html/eatingfacts.html.

Food Pyramid image: http://www.usda.gov/cnpp/pyramid.htm.

www.healthierus.gov/dietaryguidelines.

"Harvard Nutritionist says USDA 'Food Pyramid' is Wrong." http://www.rcnsc.com/general12/wrong.htm.

"MyPyramid.gov access point" (2005). United States Department of Agriculture. DGAC report, Part D. Science Base, Sect. 6. Selected Food Groups.

Reyes, R. (2008). "Food Pyramid Frenzy", *Wall Street Journal:* July 15. 2006–12.

Schlosberg, S., Neporent, L. (2005). *Fitness for Dummies.* 3rd Edition. "For Dummies" (Wiley).

U.S. Department of Health and Human Services and U.S. Department of Agriculture. Dietary Guidelines for Americans, (2005). 6th Edition. Washington, DC: U.S. Government Printing Office. Available at: http://www.mypyramid.gov/guidelines/index.html.

U.S. Department of Agriculture. MyPyramid. (2005). Available at: http://www.pyramid.gov.

Willet, W. (2005) *Eat, Drink and Be Healthy: The Harvard Medical School Guide to Healthy Eating.* Simon & Schuster.

THE NUTRIENTS

3

Nutrients are what keep us alive; they are our building blocks. Nutrients are substances found in food that help promote the growth and maintenance of our bodies. There are six essential nutrients. Remember, "essential" here means that our body cannot make them on its own, and, therefore, must obtain them through food. They are:

1. Carbohydrates
2. Lipids (chemical name for a family of fatty substances)
3. Protein
4. Vitamins
5. Minerals
6. Water

CARBOHYDRATES

Carbohydrates were discovered through the early investigations of chemists. By pouring sugar into test tubes and then burning it over a heat source, they saw that two major products were formed: water and a black substance called carbon. Thus, the name carbo (think: carbon) hydrate (think: water) was determined. The main elements making up carbohydrates are carbon, hydrogen, and oxygen. Carbohydrates are found mostly in plant based foods. Plants are able to make their own carbohydrates through a process known as photosynthesis. Photosynthesis converts energy from the sun into energy stored in carbohydrates, which the plant uses to grow. Animals are incapable of photosynthesis and must get carbohydrates from plant based foods like wheat, corn, fruits, and other vegetables. In other words, when eating bread, rice, cereal, pasta, or an apple, or broccoli, you are eating a carbohydrate.

Carbohydrates are the body's preferred energy source. In fact, they are so important, the body's central nervous system, which is composed of the brain and spine, functions solely off of carbohydrates. In other words, carbohydrates are brain fuel!

By now, almost everyone has heard of the Atkins Diet (Dr. Atkins' New Diet Revolution, 1999), which promotes weight loss through the consumption of foods low in carbohydrates and quite high in fat and protein contents, but not necessarily low in calories.

How Do These Diets Work?

You have learned that carbohydrates are crucial to central nervous system function. So, how is it that someone can consume a no-carbohydrate diet, like the Atkins' Diet? By drastically restricting carbohydrate consumption, the body goes into a different metabolic state called ketosis, where it burns its own fat and protein for fuel. When the body doesn't receive carbohydrate from its daily diet, it will start to burn protein, which is capable of being converted into a useable form of glucose (carbohydrate) to provide energy to the central nervous system. Meanwhile, fat is burned to feed other tissues and organs. However, a byproduct called ketones is produced when fat is burned without the presence of carbohydrate. This is not good! A person in ketosis is getting energy from ketones which are little carbon fragments that are the fuel created by the breakdown of fat stores. When the body is in ketosis, you tend to feel less hungry, and, as a result, you are likely to eat less than you might otherwise. Ketosis can also cause the following health problems:

Kidney Failure

Consuming too much protein puts a strain on the kidneys, which can make a person susceptible to kidney disease.

High Cholesterol

High-protein diets are typically also high in saturated fat and dietary cholesterol (consisting of red meat, whole dairy products, and other high fat foods). This type of diet is linked to high cholesterol. Studies have linked high cholesterol levels to an increased risk of developing heart disease, stroke, and cancer.

Osteoporosis and Kidney Stones

High-protein diets have been shown to cause people to excrete more calcium than normal through their urine. Over a prolonged period of time, this can increase a person's risk of osteoporosis and kidney stones.

Cancer

One of the reasons high-protein diets may increase the risks of certain health problems is because of the avoidance of carbohydrate-containing foods and the vitamins, minerals, fiber, and antioxidants they contain. It is, therefore, important to obtain your protein from a diet rich in whole grains, legumes, nuts, and low-fat dairy. Not only are you meeting your protein needs, but you are also helping to reduce your risk of developing cancer.

Ketosis

Low-carbohydrate diets can cause your body to go into a dangerous metabolic state called ketosis because your body burns fat instead of glucose for energy. During ketosis, the body forms substances known as ketones, which can cause organs to fail and result in gout, kidney stones, or kidney failure. Ketones can also dull a person's appetite, and cause nausea and bad breath. Ketosis can be prevented by eating at least 100 grams of carbohydrates a day.

In 2003 (Foster et al.), a landmark study was reported in the *New England Journal of Medicine*. The researchers conducted a controlled experiment to determine the differences in weight loss of both obese men and women who consumed either the basic low-carbohydrate Atkins Diet or a conventional diet of reduced total calories. The study lasted for one year. After three months, the volunteers who ate the Atkins Diet lost 7 to 10 percent of their original body weight, while those who ate the conventional low-calorie diet only lost 3 to 5 percent of their original weight. After six months, the results were similar to those at three months; *however,* after one year, those on the Atkins Diet had regained enough weight so that differences in weight loss between the two diets were not significant.

CARBOHYDRATE TYPES

Not all carbohydrates are created equal. Some are good for health, and some are bad and, therefore, should be limited.

There are two main categories of carbohydrates:

1. Simple
2. Complex

Simple Carbohydrates

Simple carbohydrates can be *defined* as:

Added and natural sugars

Added Sugars

Let's take a closer look at what foods contain added sugars. Added sugars are found primarily in processed foods, such as cookies, cakes, candies, sugared cereals, and sodas. In fact, most Americans are consuming more added sugar than ever before.

A United States Department of Agriculture (USDA) survey showed that sugar consumption has increased almost every year since 1982. Much of the increase is due to the consumption of soft drinks (CSPI, 1999).

The USDA advises people who eat a 2,000-calorie diet to try to limit themselves to about 10 teaspoons of added sugars per day. In fact, the average American consumes roughly 20 teaspoons of added sugars per day. Below are some examples of sugar content for common foods:

- 1 typical cup of fruit yogurt provides 70% of a day's worth of added sugar
- 1 cup of regular ice cream provides 60%
- 1 12-ounce Pepsi provides 103%
- 1 Hostess Lemon Fruit Pie provides 115%
- 1 serving of Kellogg's Marshmallow Blasted Froot Loops provides 40%
- 1 quarter-cup of pancake syrup provides 103%

Natural Sugars

Natural sugars are those found in nature. They are found in two predominant foods: fruits and dairy.

Now that we have defined simple carbohydrates (added and natural sugars), let's take a closer look at the two categories of sugars:

1. Monosaccharides
2. Disaccharides

Sugars are either a one-unit (mono) sugar or a two-unit (di) sugar. There are three **monosaccharides:**

1. *Glucose*—most simple of all sugars, major sugar found in the blood
2. *Fructose*—fruit sugar
3. *Galactose*—seldom found free in nature, part of lactose, the sugar found in milk

There are three **disaccharides,** and they each contain a glucose.

1. Glucose + Glucose = *Maltose*—sugar produced whenever starch breaks down, such as in beer production
2. Glucose + Fructose = *Sucrose*—table sugar
3. Glucose + Galactose = *Lactose*—milk sugar

It is important to recognize at this point that *both* added and natural sugars contain the same amount of calories per gram (4) because they are both types of carbohydrates. In other words, your body does *not* distinguish between the sugar in a lollipop (added) and the sugar in an apple (natural). You might then might ask, *Why do I have to limit my consumption of added sugars then?* The answer is simple: foods rich in natural sugars contain many other nutrients, like fiber, vitamins, and minerals that foods with a lot of added sugars typically do not contain. At the end of the day, a sugar is a sugar is a sugar.

For example, many people think honey is better for you than regular table sugar. Not so fast. Let's look at their chemical composition.

Table Sugar	vs.	Honey
Glucose + Fructose		Glucose + Fructose

They're the same thing! In fact, 1 teaspoon of sugar (the amount in a packet you'd get at Starbucks or Dunkin' Donuts) contains 16 calories, or 4g of carbohydrate. One teaspoon of honey, depending on the brand, contain anywhere from 25 to 40 calories! Why? Honey is highly concentrated. So, if someone is trying to lose weight, a packet of sugar at 16 calories would be preferable to a teaspoon of honey.

Complex Carbohydrates

The opposite of "simple" is "complex." Complex carbohydrates are said to be "complicated" in their chemical composition. In other words, think of a simple carbohydrate as looking like a simple wedding ring. And think of a complex carbohydrate looking like a chain-link necklace.

Two main types of complex carbohydrates exist:

1. *Starch:* Starch is defined as long chains of glucoses (monosaccharide) strung together, like the chains on a necklace.
2. *Fiber:* The indigestible portion of the plant foods that we eat.

Let's first discuss starch. Starch is technically part of a grain. There are many different types of grains such as wheat, corn, rice, barley, and oats to name a few. Grains contain three component parts with each part containing something specific. Think of an ear of corn. Now, imagine one of the kernels. This is a grain and it contains:

1. **Germ**—Tiny part of the grain containing trace amounts of oil and some vitamins and minerals. The germ is what is pressed when making some oils. For example, it takes 14 ears of corn to make 1 tablespoon of corn oil.
2. **Bran**—Rich in fiber, vitamins, and minerals.
3. **Endosperm**—Contains starch, and a little protein.

When these three component parts are in tact, the grain is referred to as a *whole grain*. Have you heard that you should try to eat more whole grains? The reason is because these grains are rich in fiber, vitamins, and minerals. Unfortunately, the grains Americans consume most are referred to as, "refined." A *refined grain* contains only the endosperm; the germ and the bran have been removed during processing. What has been lost as a result? Fiber, vitamins and minerals. In fact, a total of 22 vitamins and minerals are lost during processing.

Refined grains had a profound health impact on American health during the Great Depression. Since most people during this time struggled to afford basic necessities like food, many relied on government supplied subsidies, which included refined flour. Eating little else, many Americans began to develop deficiency diseases as a result. In an effort to solve this problem, the federal government required all refined grains to be *enriched*. An enriched grain is one that has some nutrients lost during processing replaced afterwards. In this case, the most important vitamins and minerals were put back. In fact, even today, it is the law that all refined grains contain the following four vitamins and one mineral. Take a closer look at the ingredient's list of your next food purchase. See if you can find these nutrients.

1. Folic Acid
2. Niacin
3. Thiamin
4. Riboflavin
5. Iron (only mineral)

Why Refine?

Clearly, whole grains are better for health compared to refined grains. Even though some of the lost vitamins and minerals are replaced, fiber is not replaced. You may be wondering at this point, if whole grains are so much healthier for you than refined grain, why are they refined in the first place? There are three main reasons:

1. *Longer shelf life:* Because whole grains contain a trace amount of oil, they can become rancid (spoil or rot) fairly quickly. That's why it is important to store whole grain breads in the refrigerator rather than on countertops.
2. *Profits:* A company can make more money when it breaks apart a grain. The bran can be sold as "bran flakes" cereal. The oil can be pressed into, say, corn oil. The germ can be sold as wheat germ. All of this adds up to more revenue for companies.
3. *Taste:* Most Americans are accustomed to the taste of refined grains, which make products that are fluffier and doughier in taste. Whole grains make a nuttier, denser product.

Buying Whole Grains

Finding and shopping for whole grains can be tricky. Here are some rules:

- Don't use a product's color as a guide. In other words, don't assume just because a loaf of bread is brown that it is automatically a whole grain.
- Look for the word *whole* on the package. It must say "whole" in order to be a true whole grain. For example, "100% natural stone ground wheat bread" is NOT a whole grain; however, "100% natural stone ground whole wheat bread" is.
- For rice only, you must see the word *brown*. For example, "basmati rice" is not a whole grain, but "brown basmati rice" is.
- Oats and corn are rarely refined, so even if you do not see the word whole, you can be confident that you are eating a whole grain.

Now that we've discussed starch, let's take a closer look at fiber, our second complex carbohydrate.

Fiber

Fiber is the indigestible portion of the plant foods we eat. No animal-based products contain fiber.
There are two main types of fiber:

1. Soluble fiber
2. Insoluble fiber

The term *soluble* refers to something's ability to dissolve in water. So, soluble fiber does dissolve in water while insoluble does not.

All plant foods contain *both* types of fiber. Some foods, however, contain higher amounts of one type vs. the other.

Soluble fiber binds with fatty substances in your body and helps promote their excretion as waste, thereby lowering cholesterol levels. Some foods particularly rich in soluble fiber include oats (like oatmeal), sweet potatoes, berries (like strawberries and raspberries), and legumes.

Insoluble fiber adds bulk to your fecal matter thereby speeding up the rate of your bowel movements. Foods particularly rich in insoluble fiber include corn and other whole grains.

Most Americans have no idea how many grams of fiber they get from their daily diets. Yet for many people, this number should be doubled.

A recent American Dietetic Association position paper (Marlett et al., 2002) reported that most Americans do not even come close to the recommended intake of 20 grams to 35 grams of fiber a day. Americans' mean fiber intake is about half that, about 14–15 grams a day. Children should consume their age plus 5g of fiber. So, a 5 year old should consume 10g of fiber per day (5 years old + 5 = 10g).

The amount of carbohydrate from starch and sugars that you should consume each day varies widely depending on your activity levels and goals. The 2005 Dietary Reference Intake report established acceptable macronutrient distribution ranges (AMDR) for carbohydrate. Adults and children (over 1 year old) should obtain 45 to 65 percent of their calories from carbohydrates. The wide range allows for more flexibility for people with various carbohydrate needs.

LIPIDS

Lipid is the chemical name for a family of fatty substances. There are several types of lipids such as saturated, unsaturated, and cholesterol. It is very important to understand that these are all *members* of the same family; they are not, however, all the same thing. Do not confuse saturated fat with, say, cholesterol. That would be like saying your brother or sister is the same as you because you come from the same family.

Saturated Fats

Like carbohydrates, lipids are made of carbon, hydrogen, and oxygen. Saturated fats, however, are saturated, or filled to capacity, with hydrogens. This saturation with hydrogens is what makes consuming a lot of saturated fat bad for your blood vessels and overall health.

The general rule of thumb regarding saturated fats is that they typically come from animal-based foods with the exception of coconut and palm oils, which are plant-based, and often referred to as "tropical oils." Also, they are typically solid at room temperature. If you leave a stick of butter on the kitchen counter over night, you will find the next day that it is not a liquid! It is still a solid. It is softer, but still solid.

Let's look at the food pyramid to identify where we might find a lot of saturated fat.

Bread, rice, cereal, and pasta are rich in carbohydrate and some fiber. In fact, although many people think these foods are "fattening," the reality is that they are either very low in fat or nonfat. It's not until someone adds cream cheese to a bagel, or butter to some rice or, alfredo sauce to some pasta that these foods then become fattening. Alone, however, they are very low in fat.

All fruits, with the exception of the avocado, which is technically a fruit though it is used as a vegetable in the United States, are fat-free or extremely low in fat.

All vegetables, with the exception of olives, which are pressed to make olive oil, are fat-free or extremely low in fat.

Dairy products can either be whole (full fat), low fat, or non-fat. It is important to read food labels when shopping to ensure that you buy the lowest fat version available. For example, milk in the dairy aisle can be purchased as whole milk (usually has a red cap), low fat (usually has a yellow cap), or nonfat (usually has a blue cap). Cheeses can also be purchased as full fat, low fat, or nonfat. Ultimately, dairy can either be very high fat or virtually fat free.

Meats can contain high amounts of saturated fat. Beef is like dairy in that you can purchase cuts that are high in fat or cuts that are lower in fat. Usually, cuts ending in "loin," such as sirloin or tenderloin are quite lean. Flank steak, fillet mignon, top or bottom rounds are also quite lean. Stay away from T-bone steaks, porterhouse, or other cuts with visible marbling. Marbling on a cut of steak or ground beef (the white streaks or specks you see) is all saturated fat. Chicken is quite low in fat, just avoid the skin, which is all saturated fat. White meat has less saturated fat than dark meat, however, dark meat is richer in the mineral iron than white meat. Pork can be quite lean or fatty. Bacon, sausage, and salami are all very high in saturated fat. Pork tenderloin, however, is very lean. Whatever the meat, be sure to look for fatty streaks or marbling. The more you see, the higher the saturated fat.

Beans (legumes) are very low in saturated fat. Nuts, on the other hand, are high in fat, but not saturated (see the rule above).

All seafood is fairly low in saturated fat. People find this hard to believe mostly because they associated seafood with deep frying. If you dip lobster into butter or fry shrimp in lard, it does become rich in saturated fat. But, on its own, it is quite low in saturated fat.

Unsaturated Fats

The general rule of thumb regarding unsaturated fats is that they typically come from plant-based foods with the exception of seafood, which are animal-based. Also, they are typically liquid at room temperature, like olive oil. Unsaturated fats are always preferable to saturated fats because they do not clog arteries like saturated fats do.

There are two types of unsaturated fats:

1. **Monounsaturated**—This type has one (mono) point of unsaturation (making it preferable to health). It helps increase "good" levels of blood cholesterol. Foods and oils rich in monounsaturated fats include avocado, peanuts, almonds, olive oil, canola oil, peanut oil and nut butters like peanut or almond butter.

2. **Polyunsaturated**—This type has more than one (poly) point of unsaturation (making it preferable to health). There are two types of polyunsaturated fats:

    • Linoleic fatty acid (sometimes referred to as omega-6 fatty acid): This type of polyunsaturated fat increases inflammation and blood clotting in the body. Foods and oils rich in this type of lipid include vegetable oil (which is really soybean oil), corn oil, safflower oil, sunflower oil, cottonseed oil.

    • Linolenic fatty acid (sometimes referred to as omega-3 fatty acid): This type of polyunsaturated fat decreases inflammation and blood clotting in the body. Foods and oils rich in this type of lipid include seafood especially fatty fish like tuna, salmon, halibut, and bluefish; flaxseed, tofu, and walnuts.

Note that linoleic and linolenic fatty acids act as antagonists with each other. It is best to have a *balance* of both types in your diet. The reason you may have heard that Americans should try to consume more fatty fish in their diets is because the typical American diet is especially rich in linoleic fatty acids. To balance that out, it is a good idea to eat foods rich in linolenic fatty acids, like fatty fish or other source, several times per week.

A key to understanding the different fats is remembering that whether they are good or bad for health, 1 gram of lipid contains 9 calories. In other words, do not go crazy eating "healthy" fats; they are still very high in calories!

Cholesterol

Cholesterol is a waxy substance that is often demonized, but it actually is crucial for all cellular functions in the body. It also is a key ingredient in the making of bile, which helps digest other lipids.

What is unique about cholesterol is that it is found *only in animal products.* That is because cholesterol is produced by the liver, and only animals (not plants!) have a liver. So, would peanut butter contain dietary cholesterol? Peanuts are plant-based. It is high in cholesterol's cousin, monounsaturated fat, but not cholesterol.

What is important to understand about cholesterol is that there is cholesterol we get from the foods we eat, called *dietary cholesterol.* Then, there is cholesterol that our liver produces on its own, which is often referred to as *blood serum cholesterol.* This is what your doctor measures to determine if you have high cholesterol or not. Many people still believe that eating foods high in dietary cholesterol (i.e., eggs, shrimp) are what cause you to have high blood serum cholesterol. We now know that its effect is not as strong as that of saturated fats or trans fats (DeBruyne, Pinna & Whitney, 2008).

Typically, doctors look for total cholesterol to be under 200mg/dL. Yet, we all hear about the person whose cholesterol is "normal" who has a heart attack. What is going on?

"Good" cholesterol, technically known as high density lipoprotein (HDL), is a type of cholesterol produced by the liver that helps unclog blood vessels. Eating an overall diet low in saturated and trans fats with an emphasis on unsaturated fats can help increase HDL. Vigorous exercise, as well as moderate alcohol consumption, may also help increase this good cholesterol (De Oliveira Silva *et al.,* 2000).

"Bad" cholesterol, technically known as low density lipoprotein (LDL), is a type of cholesterol produced by the liver that clogs blood vessels. Eating a diet rich in saturated and trans fats stimulates the liver to make this type of cholesterol. Why?

The bloodstream is composed mostly of water. When we eat a fat, whether it is in saturated or unsaturated form, it must be absorbed into the bloodstream from the small intestine. Herein lies the problem. The fatty blob cannot move smoothly through our watery bloodstream. To solve this transit problem, the liver is called upon to secrete lipoproteins. If you eat a lot of bad-for-you saturated and trans fats, then your liver excretes a lot of "bad" LDL cholesterol to help its transport. On the other hand, if you consume a lot of unsaturated fats, the liver is stimulated to produce more of the "good" HDL cholesterol.

Back to the heart attack patient with "normal" total cholesterol. The problem is that many Americans have "normal" cholesterol, but have disproportionate levels of HDL and LDL. Having high LDL and low HDL may make your total cholesterol appear normal.

It is best to aim for an LDL number of less than 100mg/dL. And it is ideal to have an HDL of 60mg/dL or higher.

Trans Fats

Trans fats are a man-made lipid (although a small amount of the trans fat we eat is found naturally in animal foods) that was developed in the 1980s. Around this time, consumers were looking for foods lower in fat. In response, food companies developed trans fats, also known as partially hydrogenated fats, which, at the time, were understood to be a healthier alternative to artery-clogging saturated fats. The trans fats allowed foods to still taste creamy, flaky, and crispy.

We now know that a diet containing trans fats is very unhealthy. Like saturated fat, consumption of trans fats raises LDL cholesterol (so-called "bad cholesterol") increasing your risk of heart disease. Unlike saturated fat, however, trans fat is thought to lower HDL cholesterol (so-called "good cholesterol").

A trans fat is one that begins as a healthy, unsaturated fat. It then is "hydrogenated," whereby hydrogen atoms are pumped into it replacing some of the hydrogens it was originally missing. Remember, it started off as an unsaturated fat. The result is a partially hydrogenated fat or trans fat.

These fats are found primarily in processed foods. In January 2006, the Food and Drug Administration (FDA) required all packaged foods to disclose on the nutrition facts panel how many grams of trans fat the product contained. There is a slight loop hole to this rule. A product can claim zero grams of trans fat *if* it contains less than 0.5g of trans fat per serving. Although that is a small amount of trans fat, if you eat multiple servings of foods with less than 0.5 grams of trans fat, you could exceed recommended limits. To be sure, read the ingredient's list. If you see the words *partially hydrogenated*, the product contains trans fat.

The recommended dietary allowance (RDA) for lipids is 30 percent of total calories. This 30 percent, however, should not be comprised of saturated fats. In fact, no more than 10 percent (of the 30 percent total) should come from saturated fats. Ideally, all 30 percent would come from unsaturated fat food sources. The American Heart Association (2002) recommends that no more than 1 percent of your total daily calories be trans fat. If you consume 2,000 calories a day, you should have no more than two grams of trans fat or less.

PROTEIN

Protein in food does not provide body proteins directly, but rather supply the amino acids from which the body makes its own proteins.

Protein is found in both animal, and vegetable-based foods. Animal sources include:

- Meats, like beef, pork, lamb
- Poultry, like chicken and turkey
- Dairy, like cheese, milk and yogurt
- Seafood
- Eggs

It is also found in vegetable-based sources such as:

- Legumes, like black beans and kidney beans
- Nuts, like almonds and walnuts
- Grains, like wheat (remember the endosperm?)

Proteins are made of substances known as amino acids. You can think of amino acids as being like links in a chain necklace. They string together to form a protein. Twenty different amino acids exist (DeBruyne, Pinna & Whitney, 2008) and are divided into two groups: essential and nonessential.

There are 9 essential amino acids that the body cannot make on its own and must obtain through food. There are 11 nonessential amino acids that the body *can* make on its own. In fact, the body manufactures these amino acids from the essential amino acids. If a person fails to get the 9 essential amino acids in his or her diet, then the nonessential amino acids become essential. If this happens, the amino acid is said to be "conditionally essential."

High and Low-Quality Proteins

High quality proteins provide enough of all the essential amino acids needed to support the body's work, whereas low-quality proteins do not. To determine a protein's "quality," both its amino acid composition and digestibility are taken into account. Animal-based foods (meat, fish, poultry, dairy, eggs) are considered high-quality protein sources and contain all of the essential amino acids. Protein derived from plant-based foods (legumes, nuts, and grains) tend to be limiting in one or more essential amino acids and, therefore, are considered low-quality protein sources. Soy protein, however, is one exception; it is high-quality protein just like that found in animal-based foods.

What happens if someone does not eat animal-based products? Vegans are the strictest types of vegetarians who consume *no* animal-based foods. To ensure that they are getting enough high-quality protein, they will either eat:

1. Soy-based products, such as tofu.
2. Complementary proteins, which are a combination of a grain and a legume, such as beans and rice. Each food supplies the amino acids missing in the other.

Often, when people think of protein, they think only of muscle building, but protein has other important bodily functions:

- Antibody production: Antibodies protect the body against bacteria, viruses, and other disease agents. Protein we eat helps build antibodies. In third world countries, where protein rich foods are scarce, sickness often occurs due to lack of antibody production.
- Hormone production: Protein helps build proteins, which are "chemical messengers" in the body. An example is the hormone insulin.
- Acid-base balance: Proteins also help maintain the balance between acids and bases within the body's fluids. Normal body processes constantly make acids and bases, which are carried by the bloodstream to the kidneys and lungs for excretion. The blood has to do this without upsetting the acid-base balance. Proteins act as buffers during this process helping to maintain the acid-base balance of the blood and body fluids.
- Enzyme production: Enzymes speed up chemical reactions. All enzymes are proteins. There are many different enzymes in the body that perform a range of tasks like digestion, for example.
- Growth, maintenance, and repair: The body is constantly building and repairing itself. Both inside and outside the body, cells constantly make and break down their proteins. People need to eat protein-rich foods daily to replace the protein they continually lose.

The recommended dietary allowance for protein for healthy adults is 0.8 gram per kilogram (2.2 pounds) of body weight. This results in roughly 10 percent to 35 percent of energy intake. For example:

1. Determine your body weight in pounds and then convert to kilograms (pounds divided by 2.2).
2. Multiply kilograms by 0.8 to determine total grams of protein recommended.

There are some populations that have higher-than-average protein requirements. In the United States, there is no shortage of protein in the daily diet. Yet, many people feel compelled to consume protein supplements. If too much protein is eaten, it can be stored as body fat. Also, extra protein burdens the kidneys. Athletes believe that protein shakes made with whey protein (a by-product of dairy manufacturing) will help their performance. Although whey protein may increase protein synthesis slightly, it does not appear to improve athletic performance (Tipton, 2004).

Periods of growth make protein consumption especially important for the following groups:

- Infants, children, and adolescents
- Pregnant or lactating women
- Physically active people

VITAMINS AND MINERALS

Vitamins and minerals are found in foods in tiny quantities, much smaller than the energy-yielding nutrients. Vitamins and minerals contribute no energy to the body; instead, they assist the body with most of its processes.

Vitamins fall into two categories:

1. Fat soluble
2. Water soluble

Fat Soluble

The fat-soluble vitamins dissolve in fatty substances in the body, not water. Since there is an abundance of fatty tissue in the body, these types of vitamins are particularly worrisome if taken in megadoses. Instead of the excess being excreted, as happens with water soluble vitamins, excess fat-soluble is stored in the body's fatty tissues.

There are four main fat-soluble vitamins: A, D, E, and K. To remember them, string the letters (A, D, E, K) together to form a word. ADEK sounds like the real word, *attic,* as in, you store your holiday decorations in the attic.

Vitamin A
- First fat-soluble vitamin to be recognized
- Helps overall eye health
- Prevents night blindness
- Beta-carotene: a vitamin A precursor (inactive forms of certain vitamins. Once inside the body, a precursor is converted to the active form of the vitamin). Also, an orange pigment found in fruits and vegetables like carrots.
- Acts as an antioxidant
- Good sources: fortified milk, carrots, sweet potatoes, liver, egg yolks

Antioxidants

The antioxidants are vitamins A, C, and E. String them together to help you remember them. They form the word, *ace,* like an ace bandage you would use to wrap a sprained ankle. Antioxidants act like police officers patrolling your body for substances called free radicals. Free radicals are substances that damage the body's cells. They are caused by exposure to pollutants, smoking, poor diet, and normal body processes. Antioxidants scour the body looking for these free radicals and promote their excretion as waste.

Vitamin D
- Sun exposure helps the body synthesize it on its own
- Helps the body absorb calcium important for bone health
- Good sources: egg yolks, liver, butter, some fatty fish, fortified milk

Vitamin E
- Acts as an antioxidant
- Good sources: vegetable oils, nuts, seeds

Vitamin K

- Helps with blood clotting
- Roughly 50 percent produced by bacteria in intestines
- Good sources: leafy greens like collard greens, and spinach, as well as vegetable oils like soy and canola

Water-Soluble

Water-soluble vitamins dissolve in the watery fluids of the body. Although it is difficult, it is still possible to mega-dose on these types of vitamins. Because they are water- soluble, any excess consumed is excreted through the urine as waste. That is why if you take a lot of vitamin C, for example, which is a water-soluble vitamin, you may notice that your urine is bright yellow. You are literally peeing away your money! The body excreted what it did not need. The following are the main water soluble vitamins.

Vitamin C

- Acts as an antioxidant
- Prevents scurvy, a debilitating deficiency disease that causes gums to bleed, teeth to fall out, and eventual death. Sailors on long voyages were susceptible to scurvy after perishable fruits and vegetables were consumed. Once it was determined that citrus fruits helped prevent scurvy, sailors were given lime juice to help prevent it.
- Builds collagen, which helps give elasticity to skin, ligaments, and tendons
- Good sources: citrus fruits, bell peppers, broccoli, berries

Folate

- Activates vitamin B12
- Helps synthesize DNA for new cell growth (think of a growing baby)
- Helps prevent neural tube defects like spina bifida (which literally means *open spine*)
- Good sources: leafy greens, enriched grains, beans

Vitamin B12

- Found *only* in animal-based foods, except for fortified cereals
- Activates folate
- Protects nerve cells
- Good sources: meat, poultry, fish, dairy, eggs, fortified cereals

Minerals

There are two categories of minerals: major and trace. The distinction between the major and trace minerals does not mean that one group is more important than the other. The major minerals, for example, are so named because they are needed in larger amounts by the body than the trace minerals.

Let's start with the *major minerals.*

Calcium

- Strengthens bones and teeth
- Aids muscle contraction
- Helps regulate blood pressure
- Good sources: dairy products, small fish with bones (sardines), greens like broccoli

The Electrolytes

Sodium, potassium and chloride are major minerals also known as electrolytes. Electrolytes help maintain the body's fluid balance and its acid-base balance.

Sodium
- Good sources: salt, soy sauce, process foods. The American diet is too rich in sodium resulting in hypertension.

Potassium
- All whole foods like fruits and vegetables, milk, grains, beans, and meats.

Chloride
- In addition to functioning as an electrolyte, chloride is part of the hydrochloric acid enzyme found in the stomach.
- Good sources: salt, soy sauce, processed foods

Trace Minerals

Iron
- Part of the protein hemoglobin, which carries oxygen in the blood
- Anemia is the deficiency disease associated with lack of iron
- Good sources: red meats, fish, poultry, eggs, beans, dried fruits, spinach

Iodine
- Helps thyroid function, which plays a key role in metabolic regulation.
- Good sources: iodized salt, seafood

Fluoride
- Helps make teeth resistant to decay that causes cavities
- Too much can cause fluorosis (discoloration of the teeth)
- Good sources: municipal water supplies that are fluoridated, some tea and seafood

WATER

The human body is composed of roughly 60 percent water making it an extremely vital nutrient. Every cell in the body is rich in fluid.

Functions of water in the body:
- Carries nutrients and wastes throughout the body
- Cushions and lubricates joints and bones
- Helps maintain blood pressure
- Helps maintain normal body temperature
- Helps maintain blood volume

Water intake is regulated by part of the brain known as the hypothalamus. When the blood becomes too concentrated, the mouth becomes dry and the hypothalamus signals for water to be consumed. The body must excrete about 500ml each day as urine, which is enough to carry out the waste products generated by a day's worth of metabolic activities (Debruyne, Pinna & Whitney, 2008). Water is also lost as vapor from the lungs, through fecal matter and evaporation from the skin. The general rule of thumb for water intake is to consume roughly 64 ounces, or 8 glasses, of water per day. Your first urine of the day will probably be darker yellow. If, say, by 3p.m., your urine is still dark yellow, then you are probably mildly dehydrated. Mild dehydration can cause headaches, lethargy, rapid pulse, and decreased athletic performance.

It is best to consume fluids through plain old tap or bottled water, but you can also get fluids from milk, soups, and watery fruits.

ASSIGNMENT #3

Name: _____

Date: _____

1. Look in your kitchen cabinets, bread box, pantry, and refrigerator. List foods that qualify as true, whole grains. If none do, explain what you should look for when food shopping for grains.

_____

_____

_____

_____

_____

_____

_____

_____

_____

2. Do you eat trans fats in your diet? How do you know? List the foods that you ate today. Read those with food labels, and list the food and how many grams of trans fat it contains.

_____

_____

_____

_____

_____

_____

_____

_____

_____

3. After learning more about the different nutrients, take a look at your daily diet. Which nutrients do you eat too much of? Which do you need to eat more of? Do you think you drink enough water? What are some steps you can take to improve your diet?

_____

_____

_____

_____

_____

_____

_____

_____

RESOURCES

American Heart Association: www.americanheart.org.

Atkins, R. (1999). *Dr. Atkins' New Diet Revolution.* Harper Collins: New York.

Center for Science in the Public Interest (CSPI) (1999). America: Drowning in sugar. http://www.cspinet.org/new/sugar.html.

DeBruyne, L. K., Pinna, K., Whitney, E. (2008). *Nutrition and Diet Therapy,* Seventh Edition. Thomson/Wadsworth.

De Oliveira e Silva, E. R. et al. (2000). Alcohol Consumption Raises HDL Cholesterol Levels by Increasing the Transport Rate of Apolipoproteins A-I and A-II. *Circulation;* (102) 2347–2352.

Dietary Reference Intakes for Energy, Carbohydrate, Fiber, Fat, Fatty Acids, Cholesterol, Protein, and Amino Acids (2005). *Standing Committee on the Scientific Evaluation of Dietary Reference Intakes,* page 265.

Foster, G. D., Gary D. Foster, Ph.D., Holly R. Wyatt, M. D., James O. Hill, Ph.D., Brian G. McGuckin, Ed.M., Carrie Brill, B. S., B. Selma Mohammed, M. D., Ph.D., Philippe O. Szapary, M. D., Daniel J. Rader, M. D., Joel S. Edman, D.Sc., and Samuel Klein, M. D. (2003). A Randomized Trial of a Low-Carbohydrate Diet for Obesity. *The New England Journal of Medicine:* Volume 348: 2082–2090.

Marlett, J. A., McBurney, M. I., Slavin, J. L. (2002). *Position of the American Dietetic Association: Health Implications of Dietary Fiber.* Vol. 102, Issue 7: 993–1000.

Tipton, K. D. (2004). Ingestion of casein and whey proteins result in muscle anabolism after resistance exercise. *Medicine and Science in Sports and Exercise* (36): 33–38.

DIET AND HEALTH

Leading causes of death, which include heart disease, high blood pressure, many cancers, diabetes and stroke, are largely preventable through lifestyle choices. Simple lifestyle changes can save lives and improve a person's quality of life.

Diet related diseases are linked to what we eat and kill an estimated three out of four Americans each year. These diseases include heart disease, high blood pressure, stroke, some types of cancer, and diabetes. Everyone has some degree of risk for developing diet-related chronic diseases, and this risk increases with lifestyle. Lifestyle factors that contribute to increased risk for these diseases include not eating enough fruits and vegetables, eating too many foods high in saturated fats (fried foods, full-fat dairy products, fatty cuts of meat), and not getting enough exercise.

Most Americans don't eat enough fruits and vegetables to keep them healthy. Eating a diet that contains five to nine servings of fruits and vegetables a day as part of a healthy, active lifestyle lowers the risk for all of these diseases. Calories and body weight go hand in hand with developing diet-related diseases. Excess body fat leads to an increased risk of health problems and diet-related diseases that are easily prevented through proper food intake. The earlier a person starts to eat a healthy and balanced diet, the more likely he or she will stay healthy.

The foods we eat contain a variety of vitamins, minerals, and other important nutrients that help keep our bodies healthy. All of these nutrients are needed in balanced proportion. The body cannot function properly if one or more nutrients are missing. A healthy and balanced diet provides foods in the right amounts and combinations that are safe and free from disease and harmful substances.

Food is essential for our bodies to:
- develop, replace and repair cells and tissues;
- produce energy to keep warm, move, and work;
- carry out chemical processes such as the digestion of food; and
- **protect against, resist, and fight infection and recover from sickness.**

Heart disease, which is largely influenced by what we eat, remains the number one killer of both American men and women. High blood pressure, which can be reduced within a month by changing eating habits, will affect 90 percent of American men and women at some point in their lifetime. In general, men get chronic diseases more often than women and die from them at earlier ages. African American men have even higher rates of these diseases than white men, including heart disease, high blood pressure, many cancers, and diabetes, and get them even earlier in life.

HEART DISEASE

Heart disease is a number of abnormal conditions affecting the heart and the blood vessels in the heart. Both men and women have heart attacks, but more women who have heart attacks die from them. One in three American women dies of heart disease. African American and Hispanic American/Latina women are more likely than white women to get heart disease because they tend to have more risk factors such as obesity, lack of exercise, high blood pressure, and diabetes.

Types of heart disease include:

- **Coronary artery disease (CAD)** is the most common type and is the leading cause of heart attacks. Arteries become hard and narrow. Blood has a hard time getting to the heart, so the heart does not get all the blood it needs. CAD can lead to:
  - ○ **Angina.** Angina is chest pain or discomfort that happens when the heart does not get enough blood.
  - ○ **Heart attack.** A heart attack occurs when an artery is severely or completely blocked, and the heart does not get the blood it needs for more than 20 minutes.
- **Heart failure** occurs when the heart is not able to pump blood through the body as well as it should. This means that other organs, which normally get blood from the heart, do not get enough blood.

Symptoms of a heart attack include:

- Pain or discomfort in the center of the chest
- Pain or discomfort in other areas of the upper body, including the arms, back, neck, jaw, or stomach
- Other symptoms, such as shortness of breath (feeling like you can't get enough air), breaking out in a cold sweat, nausea (feeling sick to your stomach), or feeling faint or woozy

Not everyone has all of the warning signs of heart attack. And, sometimes these signs can go away and come back.

Some women have more vague symptoms such as:

- Unusual tiredness
- Trouble sleeping
- Problems breathing
- Indigestion (upset stomach)
- Anxiety (feeling uneasy or worried)

Suggestions for reducing heart disease risk:

- **Know your blood pressure.** Your heart moves blood through your body. If it is hard for your heart to do this, your heart works harder, and your blood pressure will rise.
- **Do not smoke.** Smoking clogs your arteries.
- **Get tested for diabetes.**
- **Get your cholesterol and triglyceride levels tested.** High blood cholesterol can clog your arteries and keep your heart from getting the blood it needs. This can cause a heart attack. Triglycerides are a form of fat in your blood stream.
- **Maintain a healthy weight.** Being overweight raises your risk for heart disease.

- **Limit alcohol.** If you drink alcohol, limit it to no more than one drink (one 12 ounce beer, one 5 ounce glass of wine, or one 1.5 ounce shot of hard liquor) a day.
- **Cope with stress.** Stress hormones, such as cortisol, increase abdominal obesity and risk of heart disease.

Saturated Fat, Cholesterol, and Heart Disease

Dietary suggestions:

A diet high in saturated fat causes cholesterol, which is a soft, waxy substance, to build up in the arteries. Eventually the arteries harden and narrow. The result is an increased pressure in the arteries and a strain on the heart to maintain adequate blood flow throughout the body, which can cause a heart attack.

There are two types of cholesterol:

- **Low-density lipoprotein** (LDL) is often called the "bad" type of cholesterol because it can clog the arteries that carry blood to your heart.
- **High-density lipoprotein** (HDL) is known as "good" cholesterol because it takes the bad cholesterol out of your blood and keeps it from building up in your arteries.
- **Total cholesterol level**—Lower is better. Less than 200 mg/dL is best.

Total Cholesterol Level	Category
Less than 200 mg/dL	Desirable
200 to 239 mg/dL	Borderline high
240 mg/dL and above	High

- **LDL (bad) cholesterol**—Lower is better. Less than 100 mg/dL is best.

LDL Cholesterol Level	Category
Less than 100 mg/dL	Optimal
100–129 mg/dL	Near optimal/above optimal
130–159 mg/dL	Borderline high
160–189 mg/dL	High
190 mg/dL and above	Very high

- **HDL (good) cholesterol**—Higher is better. More than 60 mg/dL is best.
- **Triglyceride levels**—Lower is better. Less than 150mg/dL is best.

Eat foods low in saturated fats, trans fats, and cholesterol.

Eat more:
  - Fish, poultry (chicken, turkey—breast meat or drumstick is best), and lean meats (round, sirloin, loin). Broil, bake, roast, or poach foods. Remove the fat and skin before eating
  - Skim (fat-free) or low-fat (1%) milk and cheeses, and low-fat or nonfat yogurt

- ○ Fruits and vegetables (5 to 9 a day)
- ○ Cereals, breads, rice, and pasta made from whole grains (such as "whole-wheat" or "whole-grain" bread and pasta, rye bread, brown rice, and oatmeal)

Eat less:
- ○ Organ meats (liver, kidney, brains)
- ○ Egg yolks
- ○ Fats (butter, lard) and oils
- ○ Packaged and processed foods

Move more: Exercise can help lower LDL and raise HDL. Exercise at a moderate intensity for at least 30 minutes most days of the week.

Fiber and Coronary Heart Disease

The average American eats 12 grams of fiber a day; most health organizations recommend 20 to 35 grams. Studies have shown that dietary fiber clearly lower blood cholesterol. High-fiber foods are digested more slowly, so they don't cause spikes in blood-sugar levels like white bread, potatoes, and sweets do.

Some fiber, especially soluble fiber, binds to lipids such as cholesterol. The fiber then carries the lipids out of the body through the stool. This lowers the concentration of lipids in the blood and may reduce the risk of coronary heart disease.

Dietary fiber is found in plant foods, where it occurs in two forms: soluble and insoluble. Soluble fiber attracts water and turns to gel during digestion. This process slows digestion and the rate of nutrient absorption from the stomach and intestine. Soluble fiber is found in oat bran, barley, nuts, seeds, dried beans and legumes, lentils, peas, and some fruits and vegetables.

Insoluble fiber also adds bulk (fiber) to the stool. It is found in wheat bran, vegetables, and whole grains.

Soy and Lower Cholesterol

Soy has been shown to significantly lower cholesterol. The right diet can lower cholesterol as much as medication, according to a study reported July 2003 in *The Journal of the American Medical Association.* The four-week study found that a diet of soy fiber, protein from oats and barley, almonds, and margarine from plant sterols lowered cholesterol as much as statins, the most widely prescribed cholesterol medicine. Soybeans themselves provide high-quality protein, are low in saturated fat, and contain no cholesterol, making them an ideal heart-healthy food. To lower your cholesterol, the American Heart Association suggests that you look for products that provide 10 grams of soy protein per serving, and try to eat three or more servings per day. (JAMA 2003).

Antioxidants

The carotenoids and anthocyanins that provide the color for fruits and vegetables contain health-enhancing nutrients that protect against heart disease and cancer, and also improve our sense of balance, our memory, and other cognitive skills.

A Handy Guide to Antioxidants

Beta-Carotene

Found in: Orange and yellow fruits and vegetables, such as carrots and cantaloupe; dark leafy greens, such as spinach and kale.

Benefits: Beta-carotene was long believed to help prevent cataracts, although today the research appears to be more conflicted, and scientists say more research is needed.

Lutein
Found in: Leafy greens, such as spinach; corn; carrots; and squash.

Benefits: Research indicates that lutein may help lower the risk of developing cataracts and macular degeneration.

Lycopene
Found in: Red, fleshy fruits and vegetables, such as watermelon and tomatoes.

Benefits: Diets rich in lycopene may help protect against heart disease.

Selenium
Found in: Seafood, lean meats, and whole grains.

Benefits: Research often suggests that selenium may have a preventive effect against cancer.

Vitamin A
Found in: Animal sources such as eggs, meat, and dairy.

Benefits: Research indicates that vitamin A promotes clear and healthy vision. It also helps form and maintain healthy teeth, skeletal and soft tissue, and skin.

Vitamin C
Found in: Citrus fruits, such as oranges and grapefruit; bell peppers; broccoli.

Benefits: Among its many functions, vitamin C can aid tissue growth and repair, adrenal gland function, and wound repair. It may also help cure or prevent colds by boosting the immune system.

Vitamin E
Found in: Wheat germ, nuts (eg, almonds, walnuts, hazelnuts), and monounsaturated oils (eg, sunflower oil).

Benefits: Vitamin E acts as a powerful antioxidant by neutralizing free radicals in the body that cause tissue and cellular damage. Vitamin E also contributes to a healthy circulatory system and aids in proper blood clotting and improves wound healing.

American Heart Association Dietary Recommendations
- Vegetables and fruits are high in vitamins, minerals, and fiber, and low in calories. Eating a variety of fruits and vegetables may help you control your weight and your blood pressure.
- Unrefined whole-grain foods contain fiber that can help lower your blood cholesterol and help you feel full, which may help you manage your weight.
- Eat fish at least twice a week. Recent research shows that eating oily fish containing omega-3 fatty acids (for example, salmon, trout, and herring) may help lower your risk of death from coronary artery disease.

- Choose lean meats and poultry without skin and prepare them without added saturated and trans fat.
- Select fat-free, 1 % fat, and low-fat dairy products.
- Cut back on foods containing partially hydrogenated vegetable oils to reduce *trans* fat in your diet.
- Cut back on foods high in dietary cholesterol. Aim to eat less than 300 milligrams of cholesterol each day.
- Cut back on beverages and foods with added sugars.
- Choose and prepare foods with little or no salt. Aim to eat less than 2,300 milligrams of sodium per day.
- If you drink alcohol, drink in moderation, which means one drink per day if you're a woman and two drinks per day if you're a man.

HYPERTENSION (HIGH BLOOD PRESSURE)

Hypertension (high blood pressure) affects one in four adults in the United States. High blood pressure is often called the "silent killer" because it has no symptoms and can go undetected for years. Your blood pressure is the force exerted on your artery walls by the blood flowing through your body. A blood pressure reading provides two measures, systolic pressure and diastolic pressure, which are expressed as millimeters of mercury (mm Hg), or how high the pressure of blood would raise a column of mercury. Systolic pressure is measured as the heart pumps. Diastolic pressure is measured between beats, as blood flows back into the heart.

Hypertension cannot be cured, but it can be controlled through lifestyle changes and prescriptive medication. Although medications to treat hypertension are available, research has shown that modest lifestyle and dietary changes can help treat and often delay or prevent high blood pressure. Untreated hypertension causes damage to the blood vessels over time, which can lead to other health complications, such as strokes, kidney failure, impaired vision, heart attack, and heart failure.

Know Your Numbers

	Systolic (MM HG)		Diastolic (MM HG)
Normal	<120	and	<80
Prehypertension	120–139	or	80–89
HYPERTENSION			
Stage 1	140–159	or	90–99
Stage 2	≥160	or	≤100

Dietary Recommendations:

People trying to control hypertension often are advised to decrease sodium, increase potassium, watch their calories, and maintain a reasonable weight.

- The recommendation for daily sodium intake is 1,500 to 2,300 mg a day. Table salt is 40 percent sodium. One teaspoon has about 2,000 mg sodium.
- Potassium works with sodium to regulate the body's water balance. Research has shown that the more potassium and less sodium a person has in his or her diet, the greater the likelihood that the person will maintain normal blood pressure. However, the evidence does not suggest that people with high blood pressure should take potassium supplements. Instead, potassium rich foods should be eaten every-day.

- People with a low calcium intake seem to be at increased risk for hypertension. Everyone should meet the dietary reference intake (DRI) for calcium every day.
- For people who are overweight, even a small weight loss can dramatically reduce or even prevent high blood pressure.
- Incorporate the **DASH** diet into your lifestyle. A landmark study called DASH (Dietary Approaches to Stop Hypertension) looked at the effects of an overall eating plan in adults with normal to high blood pressure. Researchers found that in just eight weeks, people following the DASH diet saw their blood pressure decrease. A subsequent study called DASH 2 looked at the effect of following the DASH diet and restricting salt intake to 1,500 mg per day. Under the DASH 2 diet, people with Stage 1 hypertension had their blood pressure decrease as much or more than any anti-hypertensive medication had been able to lower it.

Strategies for Meeting the DASH diet:
- Eat more fruits, vegetables, and low-fat dairy foods.
- Cut back on foods that are high in saturated fat, cholesterol, and total fat.
- Eat more whole grain products, fish, poultry, and nuts.
- Eat less red meat and sweets.
- Eat foods that are rich in magnesium, potassium, and calcium.

The DASH Diet

Food Group	Daily Servings	Significance to the DASH Diet
Grains and grain products	7 to 8	Carbohydrates and fiber
Vegetables	4 to 5	Potassium, magnesium, and fiber
Fruits	4 to 5	Potassium, magnesium, and fiber
Low-fat or fat free milk or milk products	2 to 3	Calcium, protein, potassium, and magnesium
Meats, poultry and fish	2 or less	Protein and magnesium
Nuts, seeds and beans	4 to 5 a week	Magnesium, potassium, protein, and fiber

DIABETES

Diabetes is the sixth leading cause of death in the United States. About 65 percent of deaths among those with diabetes are attributed to heart disease and stroke. The disease often leads to blindness, heart and blood vessel disease, stroke, kidney failure, amputations, and nerve damage. Uncontrolled diabetes can complicate pregnancy, and birth defects are more common in babies born to women with diabetes.

According to recent estimates from the Centers for Disease Control and Prevention (CDC), diabetes will affect one in three people born in 2000 in the United States. The CDC also projects the prevalence of diagnosed diabetes in the United States will increase 165 percent by 2050. Diabetes prevalence in the United States is likely to increase for several reasons. First, a large segment of the population is aging. Also, Hispanics/Latinos and other minority groups at increased risk make up the fastest-growing segment of the U.S. population. Finally, Americans are increasingly overweight and sedentary. Source: http://www.cdc.gov/nccdphp/publications/aag/ddt.htm

Diabetes is a disorder of metabolism, the way our bodies use digested food for growth and energy. Most of the food we eat is broken down into glucose, the form of sugar in the blood. Glucose is the main source of fuel for the body. After digestion, glucose passes into the bloodstream, where it is used by cells for growth and energy. For glucose to get into cells, insulin must be present.

Insulin is a hormone produced by the pancreas, a large gland behind the stomach. When we eat, the pancreas automatically produces the right amount of insulin to move glucose from blood into our cells. In people with diabetes, however, the pancreas either produces little or no insulin, or the cells do not respond appropriately to the insulin that is produced. Glucose builds up in the blood, overflows into the urine, and passes out of the body in the urine. Thus, the body loses its main source of fuel even though the blood contains large amounts of glucose.

How is diabetes diagnosed?

The fasting blood glucose test is the preferred test for diagnosing diabetes in children and non-pregnant adults. It is most reliable when done in the morning.

- A blood glucose level of 126 milligrams per deciliter (mg/dL) or more after an 8-hour fast. This test is called the fasting blood glucose test.
- A blood glucose level of 200 mg/dL or more 2 hours after drinking a beverage containing 75 grams of glucose dissolved in water. This test is called the oral glucose tolerance test (OGTT).
- A random (taken at any time of day) blood glucose level of 200 mg/dL or more, along with the presence of diabetes symptoms.

The three main types of diabetes are:
- Type 1 diabetes
- Type 2 diabetes
- Gestational diabetes

Type 1 Diabetes

Type 1 diabetes is an autoimmune disease. An autoimmune disease results when the body's system for fighting infection (the immune system) turns against a part of the body. In diabetes, the immune system attacks and destroys the insulin-producing beta cells in the pancreas. The pancreas then produces little or no insulin. A person who has type 1 diabetes must take insulin daily to live.

At present, scientists do not know exactly what causes the body's immune system to attack the beta cells, but they believe that autoimmune, genetic, and environmental factors, possibly viruses, are involved. Type 1 diabetes accounts for about 5 to 10 percent of diagnosed diabetes in the United States. It develops most often in children and young adults but it can appear at any age. If not diagnosed and treated with insulin, a person with type 1 diabetes can lapse into a life-threatening diabetic coma, also known as diabetic ketoacidosis.

Symptoms may include:
- Increased thirst and urination
- Constant hunger
- Weight loss
- Blurred vision
- Extreme fatigue

Type 2 Diabetes

The most common form of diabetes is type 2 diabetes. About 90 to 95 percent of people with diabetes have type 2. About 80 percent of people with type 2 diabetes are overweight.

In type 2 diabetes, the pancreas is usually producing enough insulin, but for unknown reasons the body cannot use the insulin effectively, a condition called insulin resistance. After several years, insulin production decreases. The result is the same as for type 1 diabetes; glucose builds up in the blood and the body cannot make efficient use of its main source of fuel.

Symptoms may include:

- Fatigue
- Frequent urination
- Increased thirst and hunger
- Weight loss
- Blurred vision
- Slow healing of wounds or sores

Gestational Diabetes

Some women develop gestational diabetes late in pregnancy. Although this form of diabetes usually disappears after the birth of the baby, women who have had gestational diabetes have a 20 to 50 percent chance of developing type 2 diabetes within 5 to 10 years. Maintaining a reasonable body weight and being physically active may help prevent development of type 2 diabetes.

Gestational diabetes is caused by the hormones of pregnancy or a shortage of insulin. Women with gestational diabetes may not experience any symptoms.

Nutrition Suggestions:

Healthful eating helps keep your blood glucose, also called blood sugar, in your target range. Physical activity and, if needed, diabetes medicines also help.

Target Blood Glucose Levels for People with Diabetes

Before meals	70 to 130
1 to 2 hours after the start of a meal	less than 180

The Diabetes Food Pyramid

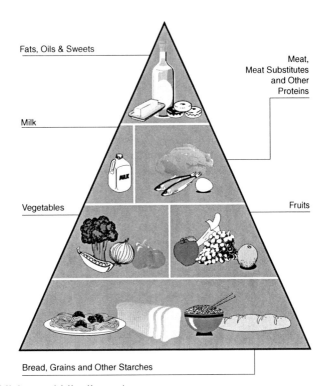

Source: Adapted from http://diabetes.niddk.nih.gov/

The diabetes food pyramid divides foods into groups, based on what they contain. A person with diabetes must eat more from the groups at the bottom of the pyramid, and less from the groups at the top. Foods from the starches, fruits, vegetables, and milk groups are highest in carbohydrate. They affect blood glucose levels the most.

Have about **1,200 to 1,600 calories** a day if you are a:

- small woman who exercises
- small or medium-sized woman who wants to lose weight
- medium-sized woman who does not exercise much

Choose this many servings from these food groups to have **1,200 to 1,600 calories** a day:	
6 starches	2 milks
3 vegetables	4 to 6 ounces meat and meat substitutes
2 fruits	up to 3 fats

Have about **1,600 to 2,000 calories** a day if you are a:

- large woman who wants to lose weight
- small man at a healthy weight
- medium-sized man who does not exercise much
- medium-sized or large man who wants to lose weight

Choose this many servings from these food groups to have **1,600 to 2,000 calories** a day:	
8 starches	2 milks
4 vegetables	4 to 6 ounces meat and meat substitutes
3 fruits	up to 4 fats

Have about **2,000 to 2,400 calories** a day if you are a:

- medium-sized or large man who exercises a lot or has a physically active job
- large man at a healthy weight
- medium-sized or large woman who exercises a lot or has a physically active job

Choose this many servings from these food groups to have **2,000 to 2,400 calories** a day:	
10 starches	2 milks
4 vegetables	5 to 7 ounces meat and meat substitutes
4 fruits	up to 5 fats

Osteoporosis

Osteoporosis is a major public health threat for 44 million Americans- 68 percent of whom are women. Osteoporosis is a disease characterized by low bone mass and structural deterioration of bone tissue, leading to bone fragility and an increased risk of fractures. Osteoporosis is a disease in which the calcium content of bones is very low. In this disease, calcium and phosphorus, which are normally present in the bones, become reabsorbed back into the body. This process results in brittle, fragile bones that are easily broken.

Throughout your lifetime, old bone is removed (resorption) and new bone is added to the skeleton (formation). During childhood and teenage years, new bone is added faster than old bone is removed. As a result, bones become larger, heavier, and denser. Bone formation outpaces resorption until peak bone mass (maximum bone density and strength) is reached around age 30.

Risk factors you cannot change:

- *Gender*—Your chances of developing osteoporosis are greater if you are a woman. Women have less bone tissue and lose bone faster than men because of the changes that happen with menopause.
- *Age*—The older you are, the greater your risk of osteoporosis. Your bones become thinner and weaker as you age.
- *Body size*—Small, thin-boned women are at greater risk.
- *Ethnicity*—Caucasian and Asian women are at highest risk. African American and Hispanic women have a lower but significant risk.
- *Family history*—Fracture risk may be due, in part, to heredity. People whose parents have a history of fractures also seem to have reduced bone mass and may be at risk for fractures.

Risk factors you can change:

- *Sex hormones*—Abnormal absence of menstrual periods (amenorrhea), low estrogen level (menopause), and low testosterone level in men can bring on osteoporosis.
- *Anorexia nervosa*—Characterized by an irrational fear of weight gain, this eating disorder increases your risk for osteoporosis.
- *Calcium and vitamin D intake*—A lifetime diet low in calcium and vitamin D makes you more prone to bone loss.
- *Medication use*—Long-term use of glucocorticoids and some anticonvulsants can lead to loss of bone density and fractures.
- *Lifestyle*—An inactive lifestyle or extended bed rest tends to weaken bones.
- *Cigarette smoking*—Cigarettes are bad for bones, as well as the heart and lungs.
- *Alcohol intake*—Excessive consumption increases the risk of bone loss and fractures.

Calcium and Osteoporosis

Dietary suggestions:

The body uses calcium to form and maintain healthy bones and teeth. Calcium also plays a vital role in nerve conduction, muscle contraction, and blood clotting. Getting enough calcium in the diet throughout childhood and puberty is one way to prevent osteoporosis.

The body's demand for calcium is greater during childhood and adolescence, when the skeleton is growing rapidly, and during pregnancy and breastfeeding. Postmenopausal women and older men also need to consume more calcium. Also, as you age, your body becomes less efficient at absorbing calcium and other nutrients. Older adults also are more likely to have chronic medical problems and to use medications that may impair calcium absorption. Add calcium-rich foods such as low-fat cheese and milk to your diet. Researchers at Purdue University found that people who consume calcium from low-fat dairy products, or get at least 1,000 milligrams a day, showed an overall decrease in body weight.

- Choose skim milk, low-fat yogurt, and low-fat cheese to avoid saturated fats. A single serving can provide you with 20 percent of the 1,200 milligrams a day you need.
- Add calcium-enriched cereals, breads, and orange juice to your diet.

- Consume foods that are dark green, leafy vegetables, such as broccoli, collard greens, bok choy, and spinach; sardines and salmon with bones; tofu; and almonds.
- Consider taking a calcium supplement.
- Add weight-bearing exercise. Like muscle, bone is living tissue that responds to exercise by becoming stronger. Weight-bearing exercise is the best for your bones because it forces you to work against gravity. Examples include walking, hiking, jogging, stair climbing, weight training, tennis, and dancing.
- Vitamin D plays an important role in calcium absorption and in bone health. It is made in the skin through exposure to sunlight. Depending on your situation, you may need to take vitamin D supplements to ensure a daily intake of between 400 to 800 IU of vitamin D.
- Give up smoking. Smoking is bad for your bones. Smokers also may absorb less calcium from their diets.
- Alcohol: Regular consumption of 2 to 3 ounces a day of alcohol may be damaging to the skeleton, even in young women and men. Those who drink heavily are more prone to bone loss and fractures, because of both poor nutrition and increased risk of falling.

Recommended Calcium Intakes (mg/day)
National Academy of Sciences

Ages	mg/day
Birth–6 months	210
6 months–1 year	270
1–3	500
4–8	800
9–13	1300
14–18	1300
19–30	1000
31–50	1000
51–70	1200
70 or older	1200
Pregnant or lactating	
14–18	1300
19–50	1000

NUTRITION FOR THE CANCER PATIENT

Half of all men and one-third of all women in the United States will develop cancer during their lifetimes. The risk of developing most types of cancer can be reduced by changes in a person's lifestyle, for example, by quitting smoking, limiting time in the sun, being physically active, and eating a better diet.

Cancer is the general name for a group of more than 100 diseases in which cells in a part of the body begin to grow out of control. Normal body cells grow, divide, and die in an orderly fashion. Cancer cells develop because of damage to DNA, which is a substance in every cell and directs all of the cell's activities. Most of the time when DNA becomes damaged, either the cell dies or is able to repair the DNA. In cancer cells, the damaged DNA is not repaired. People can inherit damaged DNA, which accounts for inherited cancers. Many times though, a person's DNA gets damaged by things in the environment, like chemicals, viruses, tobacco smoke, too much sunlight, or improper nutrition.

Because cancer cells keep growing and dividing, they are different from normal cells. Instead of dying, they outlive normal cells and continue to grow and make new, abnormal cells. Cancer usually forms as a tumor (a lump or mass.) Some cancers, like leukemia, do not form tumors; instead, these cancer cells involve the blood and blood-forming organs, and circulate through other tissues where they grow. Cancer cells often travel through the bloodstream or through the lymph system to other parts of the body where they begin to grow and replace normal tissue. This spreading process is called metastasis. Benign (non-cancerous) tumors do not spread to other parts of the body (metastasize) and are very rarely life-threatening.

Fiber and Cancer

Studies have shown that a diet high in nutrients and fiber can reduce the risk of developing cancers of the stomach, colon rectum, esophagus, larynx, and lung.

Fruits, Vegetables, and Cancer

Eating more fruits and vegetables helps provide a good supply of fiber, vitamin A, vitamin C, beta carotene and other carotenoids, and phytochemicals which are plant chemicals that may affect human health. There are hundreds of phytochemicals, and their exact role in promoting health is still unclear. However, a growing body of evidence indicates that phytochemicals may help protect against cancer.

Vitamin C and beta carotene, which forms vitamin A, are antioxidants. They protect body cells from oxidation, a process that can lead to cell damage and may play a role in cancer. Antioxidants include dark-green, leafy vegetables such as spinach, kale, collards, and turnip greens. Citrus fruits, such as oranges, grapefruit, and tangerines are also high in antioxidants. Other red, yellow, and orange fruits and vegetables—or their juices—are also healthful choices.

Alcohol and Cancer

Alcohol is processed by the liver into energy for the body. Continued and excessive use of alcohol can damage the liver in various ways, including the development of a fatty liver. A fatty liver can lead to cirrhosis of the liver. Alcohol use also increases the risk of liver cancer. When combined with smoking, alcohol intake also increases the risk of cancers of the mouth, throat, larynx, and esophagus. In addition, alcohol intake is associated with an increased risk of breast cancer in women.

Alcohol can damage the lining of the small intestine and stomach, where most nutrients are digested. As a result, alcohol can impair the absorption of essential nutrients. Alcohol also increases the body's need for some nutrients, and interferes with the absorption and storage of other nutrients.

If you choose to drink alcohol, do so in moderation. Limit yourself to no more than 2 drinks per day if male, 1 per day if female.

Nitrates and Cancer

Countries in which people eat a lot of salt-cured, smoked, and nitrite-cured foods have a high rate of cancer of the stomach and esophagus. Examples of such foods include bacon, ham, hot dogs, and salt-cured fish.

Fat and Cancer

A diet high in fat has been shown to increase the risk of cancers of the breast, colon, and prostate. A diet high in fat may promote cancer by causing the body to secrete more of certain hormones that create a favorable environment for certain types of cancer. High-fat diets also may change the characteristics of the cells to make them more vulnerable to cancer-causing agents.

To reduce fat in the diet, choose lean cuts of beef, lamb, and pork, as well as skinless poultry and fish. Baking, broiling, poaching, and steaming are recommended cooking methods. Choose skim or low-fat milk and dairy products, as well as low-fat salad dressings.

Nutrition Suggestions for People Getting Radiation Therapy

In radiation therapy, radiation is directed at the parts of the body with cancer so the cells are unable to grow and divide. People with cancer often get radiation treatments 5 days a week for 2 to 9 weeks.

The type of side effects that radiation may cause depends on the area of the body being treated, the size of the area being treated, the total dose of radiation, and the number of treatments.

Some common side effects include:

- Nausea
- Hair loss
- Fatigue
- Low blood count
- Inflammation inside the mouth
- Sensitive skin

Dietary suggestions:

- Try to eat something at least 60 minutes before treatment rather than going in with an empty stomach.
- Salty foods or ice cold drinks help control nausea.
- Avoid greasy, strong-smelling, or overly sweet foods.
- Drink plenty of water and other liquids.
- Try to eat small, frequent meals and snacks rather than three large meals and eat them slowly. If your appetite is better at certain times of the day, plan on having your largest meal then.
- Nutrition supplements, such as liquid meal replacements, can be helpful during this time.

Nutrition Suggestions for People Getting Chemotherapy

Chemotherapy involves taking strong drugs that kill cancer cells. The drugs are most commonly taken by mouth or given by injection into the bloodstream. Chemotherapy drugs can damage both healthy cells and cancer cells.

Common side effects of chemotherapy that can cause eating problems:

- Loss of appetite
- Changes in taste and smell
- Mouth tenderness or sores
- Nausea
- Vomiting

- Changes in bowel habits
- Fatigue
- Low white blood cell counts with the increased risk of infection

Dietary suggestions:
- Eat something before getting treatment.
- Eat a balanced diet that includes protein (meat, milk, eggs, and beans, lentils, and other legumes) to help boost your energy. (Chemotherapy patients are often very tired.)
- Eat small, frequent meals or snacks.
- Go easy on fried or greasy foods. These can be hard to digest.
- Drink plenty of water or liquids (eight to ten 8-oz glasses) each day.

HIV/AIDS AND NUTRITION

Good nutrition is vital to help maintain the health and quality of life of the person suffering from HIV/AIDS. When nutritional needs are not met, recovery from an illness will take longer. The HIV virus attacks the immune system. In the early stages of infection, a person shows no visible signs of illness, but later many of the signs of AIDS will become apparent, including weight loss, fever, diarrhea, and opportunistic infections (such as sore throat and tuberculosis). These infections can lower food intake because they both reduce appetite and interfere with the body's ability to absorb food. As a result, the person becomes malnourished, loses weight, and is weakened.

Food, once eaten, is broken down by digestion into nutrients. These nutrients pass through the gut walls into the bloodstream and are transported to the organs and tissues in the body where they are needed. One of the consequences of HIV, cancer and other infections is that because the gut wall is damaged, food does not pass through properly and is consequently not absorbed. When a person does not eat enough food, or the food eaten is poorly absorbed, the body draws on its reserve stores of energy from body fat and protein from muscle. As a result, the person loses weight because body weight and muscles are lost. For an average adult, serious weight loss is indicated by a 10 percent loss of body weight or 6 to 7 kg in one month.

People with HIV/AIDS often do not eat enough because:

- the illness and the medicines taken for it may reduce the appetite, modify the taste of food and prevent the body from absorbing it;
- symptoms such as a sore mouth, nausea, and vomiting make it difficult to eat; and
- fatigue, isolation, and depression reduce the appetite and the willingness to make an effort to prepare food and eat regularly.

Suggestions for gaining weight: Weight is gained by eating more food, either by eating larger portions and/or eating meals more frequently, and using a variety of foods.

- Eat more starchy foods such as rice, pasta, wheat, bread, potatoes, sweet potatoes, yams and bananas.
- Increase intake of beans, soy products, lentils, peas, groundnuts, peanut butter, and seeds, such as sunflower and sesame.
- Include all forms of meat, poultry, fish, and eggs as often as possible.
- Eat snacks regularly between meals. Good snacks are nuts, seeds, fruit, yogurt, and peanut butter sandwiches.
- Slowly increase the fat content of the food by using more fats and oils, as well as avocados.

- Introduce more dairy products.
- Add dry milk powder to foods such as porridge, cereals, sauces, and mashed potatoes.
- Add sugar, honey, jam, and syrup to the food.
- Make meals as attractive as possible.

Increase Exercise

Exercise is especially important for maintaining the health of people with HIV/AIDS. Regular exercise makes a person feel more alert, helps to relieve stress, and stimulates the appetite. Exercise is the only way to strengthen and build up muscles. The body uses muscles to store energy and protein that the immune system can draw upon when required.

ASSIGNMENT #4

Name: _____

Date: _____

Case Study

Lisa is a 46-year-old Hispanic female who is 5 feet 6 inches tall and 180 pounds. Lisa has a family history of coronary heart disease and diabetes. Two weeks ago before her doctor's appointment, a random glucose test performed with a blood glucose meter at a local health fair revealed 180 mg/dl. At the time of her appointment, routine laboratory results indicated LDL cholesterol 162 mg/dl and total cholesterol 240 mg/dl. Her triglycerides were 108 mg/dl. Her blood pressure was 140/90, and fasting blood glucose was 124.

Once an avid runner, Lisa has become less physically active in the past year, and her exercise consists of 30 minutes of low-intensity physical activity two times per week. Lisa typically eats 2 cups of frosted flakes cereal, 12 oz. of milk, and a large banana for breakfast. Her lunch consists of one ham sandwich, a Snapple iced tea, and a large fruit salad. Her main meal is a late dinner of large portions of Mexican food (such as enchiladas with rice) or lamb chops with potatoes with milk, and cookies as her late night snack. Her average daily caloric intake is approximately 2,500 kcal/day.

1. What disease(s) is Lisa at risk for and why?

_____
_____
_____
_____
_____
_____
_____
_____
_____
_____
_____
_____
_____
_____
_____
_____
_____

2. Design a plan of action for Lisa that includes a new diet, caloric expenditure, and exercise regimen. Explain why you chose the specific calories/foods/exercise for her.

_____

_____

_____

_____

_____

_____

_____

_____

_____

_____

_____

_____

_____

_____

_____

_____

_____

_____

_____

_____

_____

_____

_____

_____

_____

_____

_____

_____

_____

_____

_____

_____

_____

RESOURCES

American Cancer Society: www.cancer.org.

American Dietetic Association: www.eatright.org.

American Heart Association: www.americanheart.org.

Centers for Disease Control and Prevention: Diabetes Disabling Disease to Double by 2050: http://www.cdc.gov/nccdphp/publications/aag/ddt.htm.

DASHing to Lower Blood Pressure: www.ext.colostate.edu/PUBS/FOODNUT/09374.html.

Journal of the American Medical Association. "Effects of a Dietary Portfolio of Cholesterol-Lowering Foods vs Lovastatin on Serum Lipids and C-Reactive Protein." (2003);290(4):502–510.

Journal of the American Medical Association. "Diet First, Then Medication for Hypercholesterolemia." (2003), 290:531–533.

National Cholesterol Education Program, National Heart, Lung, and Blood Institute (NHLBI): http://www.nhlbi.nih.gov/about/ncep/.

National High Blood Pressure Education Program, National Heart, Lung, and Blood Institute (NHLBI): http://www.nhlbi.nih.gov/about/nhbpep/index.htm.

New England Journal of Medicine, "A Clinical Trial of the Effects of Dietary Patterns on Blood Pressure." (1997), 336:1117–1124.

The National Cancer Institute's CancerNet: www.cancer.gov.

The National Heart, Lung, and Blood Institute: www.www.nhlbi.nih.gov/.

The National Osteoporosis Foundation: www.nof.org.

WomenHeart: www.womenheart.org.

LIFECYCLE NUTRITION 5

In this chapter, you will gain a basic understanding of the nutritional requirements of normal healthy people over the entire lifespan incorporating the special needs of infancy and childhood, adolescence, old age, and pregnancy. You will learn the principles of nutrition assessment for different age groups, gain an understanding of the different nutrient requirements over the life cycle, and learn how the dietary recommendations for nutrient intakes are derived and applied to different populations.

INFANT NUTRITION

Food provides the energy and nutrients a baby or toddler needs to be healthy. Ensuring infants receive adequate nutrients, served in a safe and age-appropriate way, during their first year is essential to their growth and development.

For a baby, breast milk has all the necessary vitamins and minerals. Infant formulas imitate breast milk. Whenever possible, breast milk is best during the first year of life. If breast-feeding isn't possible, an iron-fortified infant formula is an acceptable alternatives. Specialized formulas are available if an infant is allergic to regular infant formulas. The baby's pediatrician can advise on the best choice. Proper formula dilution, mixing, and storage are very important. Follow directions carefully. Do not heat baby bottles in the microwave. The Centers for Disease Control and Prevention warn that children's mouths and throats can be severely burned by bottles heated in the microwave.

Nutrition Guidelines
* Children who are younger than 2 years old should obtain up to 50 percent of calories from fat.
* Whole milk is a good source of fat **after age 1.** You can switch to low-fat milk after age 2 or 3. Avoid serving regular cow's milk until infants are 1-year-old. Before then, infants may experience an allergic reaction, stomachache, and low blood iron.
* Ensure that your child gets enough iron.
* Toddlers between 1 and 3 need 500 milligrams of calcium each day.
* Dietary fiber is important after age 3 because it might prevent diseases later on in life.
* Don't feed a baby eggs, citrus fruits and juices, cow's milk, or honey until after his or her first birthday.
* Don't feed the child seafood, peanuts, or tree nuts before age 2 or 3.

- It's important to wash your hands before preparing food or formula for a baby. Not washing hands could result in infant diarrhea from the bacteria picked up by hands in the activities cited.

- Hold the baby when bottle-feeding. Babies who are put to bed with a bottle are more likely to have cavities. There is also a possibility of choking.

- The American Academy of Pediatrics (AAP) recommends giving juice only to infants who are approximately 6 months or older and who can drink from a cup. AAP recommends offering no more than a total of 4 to 6 ounces of juice a day to infants.

- Do not serve infants honey or corn syrup during the first year of life. These foods may contain botulism spores which could cause illness or death in infants.

- AAP recommends breast milk or a prepared iron-fortified infant formula be the only nutrient fed to infants until 4 to 6 months of age.

- When introducing new foods, try only one at a time and start with single-ingredient foods. Avoid serving mixed ingredient foods until each food has been given separately so you can tell if a baby is allergic to a specific food. Begin by serving about 1 to 2 tablespoons and then increase the amount as baby wants more. Wait a week before trying another new food so you identify any allergic reactions to it.

- Iron-fortified rice cereal is usually the first cereal offered, as babies are least likely to be allergic to it. It's frequently recommended to continue fortified baby cereal through the first year of life.

- Infants may be allergic to egg whites.Wait until about 12 months before offering this food. They may be able to tolerate egg yolks around 8 months.

- Avoid feeding directly from the baby food jar. Bacteria from a baby's mouth can grow and multiply in the food before it is served again. Too many bacteria can make a baby sick. Refrigerate food remaining in the jar and use within 1 to 2 days after opening.

- Do not heat baby foods in their original containers in the microwave. The heat is uneven and can produce "hot spots" that can scald a baby's mouth and throat. Also, the food in the jar may "blow up" in your microwave.

- Once food is opened, don't leave baby food solids or liquids at room temperature for more than 2 hours. Bacteria can grow to harmful levels when food is left out longer than this.

- Avoid serving foods that may choke an infant, such as nuts and seeds, raw carrots and celery, whole kernel corn, raisins, large chunks of meat or cheese, popcorn, chips, pretzels, adult dry cereal, grapes, berries, cherries, unpeeled fruits and vegetables, hard candies, pickles, hot dogs, marshmallows (regular or miniature), and peanut butter. In general, avoid foods that are round and firm, sticky, or cut in large chunks.

TODDLER NUTRITION

Babies grow at a lightning pace 3 inches (8 centimeters) or so every 3 months. A toddler, in contrast, grows at a much slower rate only 3 to 5 inches (8 to 13 centimeters) in an entire year.

The toddler years are a time of transition, especially between 12 to 24 months, when they're learning to eat table food and accepting new tastes and textures. Depending on their age, size, and activity level, toddlers need about 1,000 to 1,400 calories a day. Fat intake should not be restricted in an infant's diet, but by age 2, a toddler should get only 30 to 35% of daily calories from fat.

Calcium

Children under age 2 should have whole milk to help provide the dietary fats that they need for normal growth and brain development. After age 2, most children can switch to low-fat or nonfat milk. Toddlers should have 500 milligrams of calcium a day. This requirement is easily met if a child gets the recommended two servings of dairy foods every day. An important part of a toddler's diet, milk provides calcium and vitamin D to help build strong bones. Some children don't like milk or are unable to drink or eat dairy products. Explore other calcium sources, such as fortified cereals, calcium-fortified soy beverages, broccoli, and calcium-fortified orange juice.

Drinking a lot of cow's milk (more than 24 to 36 ounces/720 milliliters) also can put a child at risk of developing iron deficiency. Toddlers who drink a lot of cow's milk may be less hungry and less likely to eat iron-rich foods. Milk decreases the absorption of iron and can also irritate the lining of the intestine, causing small amounts of bleeding and the gradual loss of iron in the stool.

Iron

Iron deficiency can affect growth and may lead to learning and behavioral problems and anemia (a decreased number of red blood cells in the body). Iron is needed to make red blood cells, which carry oxygen throughout the body. Without enough iron and red blood cells, the body's tissues and organs get less oxygen and do not function as well.

Toddlers should have 7 milligrams of iron each day. After 12 months of age, toddlers are at risk for iron deficiency because they no longer drink iron-fortified formula and may not be eating iron-fortified infant cereal or enough other iron-containing foods to make up the difference.

To help prevent iron deficiency:

- Limit a child's milk intake to about 16 to 24 ounces (480 to 720 milliliters) a day.
- Serve more iron-rich foods (meat, poultry, fish, enriched grains, beans, tofu).
- When serving iron-rich meals, include foods that contain vitamin C (tomatoes, broccoli, oranges, and strawberries), which improve the body's iron absorption.
- Continue serving iron-fortified cereal until the child is 18 to 24 months of age.

Nutrition Guidelines for Toddlers

Food Group	Daily Amount for 2-Year-Olds	Daily Amount for 3-Year-Olds	Servings
Grains	3 ounces (85 grams), half from whole-grain sources	4 to 5 ounces (110 to 140 grams), half from whole-grain sources	One ounce equals: 1 slice bread 1 cup of ready-to-eat cereal, or ½ cup of cooked rice, cooked pasta, or cooked cereal
Vegetables	1 cup	1.5 cups	Serve vegetables that are soft, cut in small pieces, and well cooked to prevent choking
Fruits	1 cup	1 to 1 ½ cups	An 8 to 9 inch (20 to 23 centimeter) banana equals 1 cup
Milk	2 cups (475 milliliters)	2 cups (475 milliliters)	One cup equals: 1 cup of milk or yogurt, 1 ½ ounces (45 grams) of natural cheese, or 2 ounces (60 grams) of processed cheese
Meat & Beans	2 ounces (60 grams)	3 to 4 ounces (85–115 grams)	One ounce equals: 1 ounce (30 grams) of meat, poultry or fish, ¼ cup cooked dry beans, or 1 egg

CHILD/ADOLESCENT NUTRITION

A healthy diet helps children grow and learn. It also helps prevent obesity and weight-related diseases, such as diabetes. Children who are overweight are more likely to develop type 2 diabetes, high blood pressure, heart disease, and other illnesses that can follow them into adulthood. Obesity in children can also lead to stress, sadness, and low self-esteem.

As children spend more time watching television and playing computer and video games, they spend less time being active. Parents play a big role in helping kids get up and get moving. Experts suggest at least 60 minutes of moderate physical activity daily for most children.

Research has shown that children who skip breakfast do not do as well in school as students who eat breakfast. A healthy breakfast includes a whole grain cereal, oatmeal, or bread with a protein such as peanut butter or a hard-boiled egg. Including whole fruit instead of fruit juice adds more vitamins, minerals, and fiber into the diet. Dairy products are acceptable as long as they are in the form of fat-free or low-fat milk, yogurt, or cheese.

When children consume a high-fat, high-sugar meal, their bodies will crash. They will become very tired and lethargic, which is not going to help them perform in school.

Lunches should include a type of whole grain, such as bread or tortillas, with a lean protein, such as tuna, turkey, or chicken. Include assortments of fruits and vegetables in various colors and sizes. Healthy beverage choices include water, fat-free or low-fat milk, or 100-percent fruit juice.

At dinner, half of a child's plate should include vegetables and fruit, one-quarter should consist of a lean protein, and one-quarter should contain whole grains, such as brown rice or whole wheat pasta.

Nutrition Guidelines for Children/Adolescents

- Offer five servings of fruits and vegetables a day.
- Choose healthy sources of protein, such as lean meat, nuts, and eggs.
- Serve whole-grain breads and cereals because they are high in fiber.
- Broil, grill, or steam foods instead of frying them.
- Limit fast food and junk food.
- Offer water and milk instead of sugary fruit drinks and sodas.
- Serve calcium-rich vegetables like broccoli, mustard greens, kale, collard greens, and brussel sprouts.
- Cook with less fat. Bake, roast, or poach foods instead of frying.
- Limit the amount of added sugar in a child's diet.
- Serve water or low-fat milk more often than sugar-sweetened sodas and fruit-flavored drinks.
- Involve the child in planning and preparing meals. Children may be more willing to eat the dishes that they help fix.
- Parents should serve as role models for their children. If children see their parents being physically active, they are more likely to be active and stay active throughout their lives.

TEEN NUTRITION

Teens may feel stressed from school, after-school activities, peer pressure, and family relationships. Many have busy schedule, that lead them to skip breakfast, buy lunch from vending machines, and grab whatever is in the refrigerator for dinner.

Healthy behaviors, like nutritious eating and regular physical activity, may help teens meet the challenges of their stressful lives. Healthy eating and regular exercise may help them feel energized, learn better, and stay alert in class. These healthy habits may also lower risks for diseases such as diabetes, asthma, heart disease, and some forms of cancer.

Many teens turn to unhealthy dieting methods to lose weight, including eating very little, cutting out whole groups of foods (like grain products), skipping meals, and fasting. Other weight-loss tactics such as smoking, self-induced vomiting, or using diet pills or laxatives can lead to health problems. Unhealthy dieting can actually cause weight gain because it slows down the metabolism.

Nutrition Guidelines for Teens

- Eat fruits and vegetables every day. Teenagers who are consuming 2,000 calories per day should aim for 2 cups of fruit and 2-½ cups of vegetables every day.
- Calcium helps strengthen bones and teeth. Calcium is very important, because getting enough calcium now can reduce the risk for broken bones later in life. Aim for at least three 1 cup-equivalents of low-fat or fat-free calcium-rich foods and beverages each day.
- Protein builds and repairs body tissue, like muscles and organs. Eating enough protein can help you grow strong and sustain your energy levels. Teens need five and one-half 1 ounce-equivalent of protein-rich foods each day.
- Whole-grain foods like whole-wheat bread, brown rice, and oatmeal usually have more nutrients than refined grain products. They give you a feeling of fullness and add bulk to your diet. Try to get six 1 ounce-equivalents of grains every day, with at least three 1 ounce-equivalents coming from whole-grain sources. They are also a great energy source.
- Get iron. Teen boys need iron to support their rapid growth. Most boys double their lean body mass between the ages of 10 and 17. Teen girls also need iron to support growth and replace blood lost during menstruation.

To get the iron they need, teens should eat the following foods:

- Fish and shellfish
- Lean beef
- Iron-fortified cereals
- Enriched and whole-grain breads
- Cooked dried beans and peas like black beans, kidney beans, black-eyed peas, and chickpeas/garbanzo beans
- Spinach
- Fat helps the body to grow and develop. Fat is a source of energy as well; it even keeps the skin and hair healthy. Limit your fat intake to 25 to 35 percent of your total calories each day. Limit saturated fat and trans fat, which can clog your arteries and raise your risk for heart disease. Look for words like "*shortening,*" "*partially hydrogenated vegetable oil,*" or "*hydrogenated vegetable oil*" in the list of ingredients.

Healthier fat sources include:

- Olive, canola, safflower, sunflower, corn, and soybean oils
- Fish like salmon, trout, tuna, and whitefish
- Nuts like walnuts, almonds, peanuts, and cashews

Saturated fat is found primarily in:

- Butter
- Full-fat cheese
- Whole milk
- Fatty meats
- Coconut, palm, and palm kernel oils

Trans fat is often found in:
- Baked goods, like cookies, muffins, and doughnuts
- Snack foods, like crackers and chips
- Vegetable shortening
- Stick margarine
- Fried foods

Limit fast food and choose wisely. If you do order fast food, try these tips:
- Skip "value-sized" or "super-sized" meals.
- Choose a grilled chicken sandwich or a plain, small burger.
- Use mustard instead of mayonnaise.
- Limit fried foods or remove breading from fried chicken, which can cut half the fat.
- Order garden or grilled chicken salads with light or reduced-calorie dressings.
- Choose water, fat-free, or low-fat milk instead of sweetened soda.

Research has shown that being physically active may:
- Help you control your weight, build lean muscle, and reduce your body fat.
- Strengthen your bones.
- Increase flexibility and balance.
- Reduce your risk for chronic diseases like type 2 diabetes, heart disease, and high blood pressure.
- Improve your self-esteem and mood.
- Decrease feelings of anxiety and depression.
- Help you do better in school.

Female Athlete Triad Syndrome

Girls who play sports are healthier; get better grades; are less likely to experience depression; and use alcohol, cigarettes, and drugs less frequently than girls who aren't athletes. Some girls who play sports or exercise intensely are at risk for a problem called female athlete triad. Female athlete triad is a combination of three conditions: disordered eating, amenorrhea, and osteoporosis. A female athlete can have one, two, or all three parts of the triad.

Triad Factor #1: Disordered Eating

Most girls with female athlete triad try to lose weight primarily to improve their athletic performance. The disordered eating that accompanies female athlete triad can range from avoiding certain types of food the athlete thinks are "*bad*" (such as foods containing fat) to serious eating disorders like anorexia nervosa or bulimia nervosa.

Triad Factor #2: Amenorrhea

Because a girl with female athlete triad is simultaneously exercising intensely and not eating enough calories, when her weight falls too low, she may experience decreases in estrogen, the hormone that helps to regulate the menstrual cycle. As a result, a girl's periods may become irregular or stop altogether.

Triad Factor #3: Osteoporosis

Low estrogen levels and poor nutrition, especially low calcium intake, can lead to osteoporosis. Usually, the teen years are a time when girls should be building up their bone mass to their highest levels, called peak bone mass. Osteoporosis is a weakening of the bones due to the loss of bone density and improper bone formation. Not getting enough calcium during the teen years can also have a lasting effect on how strong a girl's bones are later in life.

Signs and Symptoms of Triad Syndrome

- Weight loss
- No periods or irregular periods
- Fatigue and decreased ability to concentrate
- Stress fractures
- Muscle injuries

Signs and Symptoms of Eating Disorders

- Continued dieting in spite of weight loss
- Preoccupation with food and weight
- Frequent trips to the bathroom during and after meals
- Use of laxatives
- Brittle hair or nails
- Dental cavities (with bulimia, tooth enamel is worn away by frequent vomiting)
- Sensitivity to cold
- Low heart rate and blood pressure
- Heart irregularities and chest pain

Self-Esteem and Body Image

Self-esteem is all about how much people value themselves, the pride they feel in themselves, and how worthwhile they feel. Self-esteem is important because feeling good about yourself can affect how you act. A person who has high self-esteem will make friends easily, is more in control of his or her behavior, and will enjoy life more.

Body image is how a person feels about his or her own physical appearance.

Some teens struggle with their self-esteem and body image when they begin puberty because the body goes through many changes. Girls may feel pressure to be thin, and guys may feel like they don't look big or muscular enough. Other factors like media images can affect a person's body image too. Family life can sometimes influence a person's self-esteem. Some parents spend more time criticizing their children and the way they look than praising them. This criticism may reduce a person's ability to develop good self-esteem. People may also experience negative comments and hurtful teasing about the way they look from classmates and peers.

Healthy Self-Esteem and Body Image

If you have a positive body image, you probably like and accept yourself the way you are. Some people think they need to change how they look or act to feel good about themselves. In reality all you need to do is change the way you see your body and how you think about yourself.

The first thing to do is recognize that your body is your own, no matter what shape, size, or color it comes in. Next, identify which aspects of your appearance you can realistically change and which you can't. Everyone- (even the most perfect-seeming celeb)- has things about themselves that they can't change and need to accept, like their height, or their shoe size for example.

If there are things about yourself that you want to change and can (such as how fit you are), do this by making goals for yourself. Then keep track of your progress until you reach your goal.

When you hear negative comments coming from within yourself, tell yourself to stop. Try building your self-esteem by giving yourself compliments every day. By focusing on the good things you do and the positive aspects of your life, you can change how you feel about yourself.

Resilience is the number one skill that increases self-esteem. People who believe in themselves are better able to recognize mistakes and bounce back from disappointment.

PREGNANCY

What you eat right before and during your pregnancy can affect the health of your growing baby. Even before you start trying to get pregnant, you should take special care of your health.

Getting enough folic acid is most important very early in pregnancy, usually *before* a woman knows she is pregnant. Folic acid is a B vitamin that helps prevent serious birth defects of a baby's brain or spine, called neural tube defects. Getting enough folic acid can also help prevent birth defects like cleft lip and congenital heart disease. Some breakfast cereals are enriched with 100% of the folic acid that your body needs every day.

While you are pregnant, you will need additional nutrients to keep you and your baby healthy. That does not mean, however, you need to eat twice as much. According to the American Dietetic Association (ADA), a pregnant woman needs only 300 calories a day more than she did pre-pregnancy. The ADA recommends that pregnant women eat a total of 2,500 to 2,700 calories every day.

Make sure not to restrict your diet during pregnancy either. If you do, your unborn baby might not get the right amounts of protein, vitamins, and minerals. Low-calorie diets can break down a pregnant woman's stored fat, which can lead to the production of substances called ketones. Constant production of ketones can result in a mentally retarded child.

Nutrition Guidelines during Pregnancy

- **Fruits and vegetables.** Pregnant women should try to eat 7 or more servings of fruits and vegetables combined (for example, 3 servings of fruit and 4 of vegetables) daily.
- **Whole-grains or enriched breads/cereals.** Pregnant women should eat 6 to 9 servings of whole-grain or enriched breads and/or cereals every day.
- **Dairy products.** Pregnant women should try to eat 4 or more servings of low-fat or non-fat milk, yogurt, cheese, or other dairy products every day.
- **Proteins.** Pregnant women and their growing babies need 10 grams of protein more than non-pregnant women. Pregnant women should eat 60 grams of protein every day. Two or more 2 to 3 ounce servings of cooked lean meat, fish, or poultry without skin, or two or more 1 ounce servings of cooked meat contain about 60 grams of protein. Eggs, nuts, dried beans, and peas also are good sources of protein.
- **Don't eat uncooked or undercooked meats or fish.** These can make you sick and may harm your baby. Pregnant women should also avoid deli luncheon meats.
- **Folic acid.** Pregnant women need 400 micrograms (400 mcg) of folic acid every day to help prevent birth defects.
- **Iron.** Pregnant women need twice as much iron-30 mg per day- than other women. Some good sources of iron include lean red meat, fish, poultry, dried fruits, whole-grain breads, and iron-fortified cereals. Pregnant women need extra iron for the increased amount of blood in their bodies. Iron helps keep your blood healthy.
- **Water.** Pregnant women should drink at least six eight-ounce glasses of water per day. Plus, pregnant women should drink another glass of water for each hour of activity. Drinking enough water, especially in your last trimester, prevents you from becoming dehydrated. Not getting enough water can lead to premature or early labor. It also helps prevent constipation, hemorrhoids, excessive swelling, and urinary tract or bladder infections.

- **Fish and shellfish.** Fish and shellfish are a great source of protein and heart-healthy omega-3 fatty acids. But almost all fish and shellfish contain a harmful substance called mercury. Mercury mainly gets into our bodies by the fish we eat. High levels of this metal seem to be harmful to developing babies.
  - Do not eat any shark, swordfish, king mackerel, or tilefish (also called golden or white snapper).
  - Do not eat more than six ounces of "white" or "albacore" tuna or tuna steak each week.
  - Choose shrimp, salmon, pollock, catfish, or "light" tuna because they contain less mercury.
- **Weight gain.** The American College of Obstetricians and Gynecologists (ACOG) recommends an average weight gain of 25 to 30 pounds during pregnancy. The amount of weight you should gain, however, depends on your weight before you became pregnant and your height.
  - If you were underweight before becoming pregnant, you should gain between 28 and 40 pounds.
  - If you were overweight before becoming pregnant, you should gain between 15 and 25 pounds.
  - You should gain weight gradually during your pregnancy, with most of the weight gained in the last trimester.
- **Fetal alcohol spectrum disorders (FASD)** is a term describing a range of effects that can occur in a person whose mother drank alcohol during pregnancy. Some people with FASD have abnormal facial features and growth and central nervous system problems. People with FASD may have problems with learning, memory, attention span, communication, vision, and/or hearing. These problems often lead to problems in school and social problems. There is no safe time during pregnancy for you to drink alcohol. There is no known safe amount of alcohol to drink during pregnancy.

Caffeine is a stimulant found in colas, coffee, tea, chocolate, cocoa, and some over-the-counter and prescription drugs. Large quantities of caffeine can cause irritability, nervousness, and insomnia, as well as low birth-weight babies and miscarriages. Caffeine is also a diuretic and can rob the body of valuable water. Some studies show that drinking caffeine during pregnancy can harm the fetus. Other research suggests that small amounts of caffeine are safe.

NUTRITION FOR OLDER ADULTS

People in the United States are living longer than ever before. Many older adults live active and healthy lives. Eating a balanced diet, keeping mind and body active, not smoking, getting regular checkups, and practicing safety habits will help you make the most of life. Studies show that a good diet in your later years reduces your risk of osteoporosis, high blood pressure, heart disease, and certain cancers.

Older people eventually face one or more problems that interfere with their ability to eat well. Social isolation is a common one. Older people who find themselves single after many years may become depressed and lose interest in preparing or eating regular meals, or they may eat only sparingly.

Chronic medical problems require many older adults to follow special diets such as a low-fat, low-cholesterol diet for heart disease, a low-sodium diet for high blood pressure, or a low-calorie diet for weight reduction. Special diets often require extra effort, but older people may instead settle for foods that are quick and easy to prepare, such as frozen dinners, canned foods, lunch meats, and others that may provide too many calories, or contain too much fat and sodium for their needs. Adverse reactions from medications can cause older people to avoid certain foods. Some medications alter the sense of taste, which can adversely affect appetite. Dementia associated with Alzheimer's and other diseases may cause older adults to eat poorly or forget to eat altogether.

Some older people have chewing difficulties and gastrointestinal disturbances, such as constipation, diarrhea, and heartburn. Because missing teeth and poorly fitting dentures make it hard to chew, older people may forego fresh fruits and vegetables, which are important sources of vitamins, minerals, and fiber. Or they may avoid dairy products, believing they cause gas or constipation. By doing so, they miss out on important sources of calcium, protein, and some vitamins.

Lack of money is a particular problem among older Americans, who may have no income other than Social Security. Lack of money may lead older people to scrimp on important food purchases—for example, perishable items like fresh fruits, vegetables, and meat-because of higher costs and fear of waste.

Nutrition Guidelines for Older Adults

Researchers from Tufts University developed a Food Guide Pyramid to more accurately represent the calorie and special nutrient needs for healthy persons over the age of 70.

- Eat at least the minimum number of servings for each food group in the Food Guide Pyramid. Eat a variety of foods that are good sources of protein, vitamins, minerals, and fiber.
- Eat at least three servings of calcium-rich foods. Calcium and vitamin D are important to maintain bone health.
- Drink 8 cups of water as the base of the 70+ Pyramid. This is needed because of higher intake of medications and to prevent dehydration and constipation.
- Eat fiber-rich foods from grains, fruits, vegetables, dried beans, and nuts.
- Eat fortified foods with vitamin B12, calcium, and vitamin D.
- Avoid empty calories, which are foods with lots of calories but few nutrients, such as chips, cookies, soda, and alcohol.
- Pick foods that are low in cholesterol and fat, especially saturated and trans fats.

Physical activity can help reduce and control weight by burning calories. Moderate exercise that places weight on bones, such as walking, helps maintain and possibly even increases bone strength in older people. A study published in the Dec. 28, 1994, *Journal of the American Medical Association* found that intensive strength training can help preserve bone density and improve muscle mass, strength, and balance in postmenopausal women. In the study, subjects used weight machines for strength training. Regular exercise can improve the functioning of the heart and lungs, increase strength and flexibility, and contribute to a feeling of well-being.

ASSIGNMENT #5

Name: _____

Date: _____

1. Pick a person to interview from one of the lifecycle categories discussed in this chapter. The interview should consist of some of the below questions or original questions.

2. Describe this person and report on their daily nutritional and exercise habits.

3. Using the nutritional suggestions in this chapter, guide them into changing their nutrition and exercise habits. Report on this process.

Possible Interview Questions

- Describe a typical day of eating. Include amounts and location of where food is eaten or purchased.
- Do you exercise on a regular basis?
- Is your kitchen stocked with fruits; vegetables; low-fat or fat-free milk, and milk products; whole-grain items; and other foods you need to eat healthy?
- Can you get water and low-fat or fat-free milk instead of soda, sweetened tea, and sugary fruit drinks?
- Do you pack healthy lunches to take to school or work?
- Does your family eat dinner together a few times per week?
- How many hours do you spend watching television or playing video or computer games?
- Does the cafeteria offer healthy foods such as salads and fruit?
- Are there vending machines at school or work where you buy snacks and drinks?

_____
_____
_____
_____
_____
_____
_____
_____
_____
_____
_____
_____
_____
_____
_____
_____
_____

RESOURCES

Administration on Aging: www.aoa.gov/eldfam/eldfam.asp.

American Academy of Pediatrics Committee on Nutrition. (2001). "The Use and Misuse of Fruit Juice in Pediatrics." *Journal of Pediatrics*. 107:1210–1213.

American Academy of Pediatrics: www.aap.org/parents.html.

American College of Obstetricians and Gynecologists: http://www.acog.org.

American Dietetic Association. (1998). *Staying Healthy-A Guide for Older Adults*. Chicago: The American Dietetic Association.

American Dietetic Association: www.eatright.org.

Dietary Guidelines for Americans. USDA and DHHS, 2005: www.healthierus.gov/dietaryguidelines.

Food and Nutrition Information Center, USDA; Agricultural Research Service: www.nal.usda.gov/fnic.

International Food Information Council: http://ific.org.

Journal of the American Medical Association. (1994). "Effects of high-intensity strength training on multiple risk factors for osteoporotic fractures. A randomized controlled trial." Dec 28; 272(24):1909–14.

Konikoff, R. A. (March, 1999). A modified food guide for people over 70 years. *Nutritional commentator*, Tufts University.

President's Council on Physical Fitness and Sports: www.fitness.gov.

Schlenker, E. D. (1998). Nutrition in aging. 3rd ed. Boston: McGraw-Hill.

The National Network for Child Care: www.nncc.org.

WeCan! Ways to Enhance Children's Activity and Nutrition: wecan.nhlbi.nih.gov.

Weight-control Information Network: www.niddk.nih.gov.

RESOURCE WEB-SITES

www.mypyramid.gov is your access point for the U.S. Department of Agriculture's (USDA) food guidance system. This website contains general guidance on food and healthy eating, with tips and suggestions for making smart dietary choices. The site also features interactive tools that can customize food and calorie recommendations according to your age, gender, and physical activity level.

www.fitness.gov, run by The President's Council on Physical Fitness and Sports, provides regular updates on the Council's activities as well as resources on how to get involved in its programs.

www.girlshealth.gov, developed by the Office on Women's Health, provides girls with reliable health information on physical activity, nutrition, stress reduction, and more.

www.fns.usda.gov/tn is the USDA's Team Nutrition website, which focuses on the role nutritious school meals, nutrition education, and a health-promoting school environment play in helping students learn to enjoy healthy eating and physical activity.

www.nichd.nih.gov/msy is the National Institute of Child Health and Development's *Media-Smart Youth: Eat, Think, and Be Active!* program. This interactive after-school program is designed to help young people become aware of the media's influence on their food and physical activity choices.

www.cdc.gov/powerfulbones is part of the Centers for Disease Control and Prevention's (CDC) *Powerful Bones, Powerful Girls*, which is a national health campaign that provides tips on healthy eating and physical activity.

www.canfit.org, the website of the California Adolescent Nutrition and Fitness Program, provides resources on adolescent nutrition and body image, fitness, and more.

http://hin.nhlbi.nih.gov/portion/keep.htm is a quiz from the National Heart, Lung, and Blood Institute that tests your knowledge of how food portion sizes have changed during the last 20 years.

www.cdc.gov/nccdphp/dnpa/physical/index.htm, a site sponsored by the CDC's Division of Nutrition and Physical Activity, addresses the importance of physical activity and provides recommendations on how to get started on a fitness program. It includes links to websites that offer health information for teenagers.

NUTRITIONAL TRENDS 6

Several prominent nutritional trends are influencing consumers to buy certain foods or follow certain eating plans. This chapter will highlight some of the trendy eating plans or "diets" consumers are trying now, as well as other trends that have gained a loyal following.

ORGANIC FOOD

Organic food is produced according to certain production standards. Simply put, it is grown without the use of conventional pesticides, artificial fertilizers, human waste, or sewage sludge, and it is processed without ionizing radiation or food additives. Livestock are reared without use of antibiotics and without the use of growth hormones.

The term *natural* does not mean organic. Unfortunately, consumers confuse the two terms. Natural can refer to one or more ingredients derived from a plant or animal that's added for flavor, not nutrition. For example, mint ice cream may contain "natural flavor," in reference to the peppermint added.

Organic food production is legally regulated. Currently, the European Union, the United States, Canada, Japan, and many other countries require producers to obtain organic certification to market food as organic. Organic products are now marketed in major supermarkets across the United States, and the industry is experiencing significant annual growth.

Although most of us think of milk or eggs as being available as organic, the "organic" category now includes foods like wine, and caviar. The combination of significant mass marketing and health-conscious consumers who favor foods without synthetic herbicides, pesticides or hormones, has caused organic foods to skyrocket. In fact, in 2004, retail sales of organic foods exceeded $15 billion with more than $32 billion projected by 2009 (Hansen, 2004).

What to Look For

When buying organic foods, look for the "USDA Organic" seal. Only foods in the categories of "100% organic" and "organic" may display the USDA Organic seal. The following are definitions according to the National Organic Program of the USDA (2003).

- *100% organic:* Single ingredient such as a fruit, vegetable, meat, milk and cheese (excludes water and salt).
- *Organic:* Multiple ingredient foods that are 95% to 100% organic.
- *Made with organic ingredients:* 70% of the ingredients are organic.
- *Contains organic ingredients:* Contains less than 70% organic ingredients.

Many people believe that organic food is more expensive, which, in general, is accurate. Organic food costs more than conventional food because of the laborious and time-intensive systems used by the typically smaller organic farms; however, the benefits of buying organic may off-set this additional cost. Consider the following points when questioning the price of organic (www.organic.org):

- Organic farmers do not receive federal subsidies like conventional farmers do; therefore, the price of organic food reflects the true cost of growing.
- The price of conventional food does not reflect the cost of environmental cleanups that we pay for through our tax dollars.
- Organic farming is more labor and management intensive.

Why Organic?

Today's consumer often wonders if buying organic really means anything and if it is financially "worth" it, especially given all the news about rising food costs in general. Organic food is more expensive, but when it comes to the staples of your diet, organics are a worthwhile investment, with payoffs that might surprise you.

Organic Food Has More Nutrients

There are reasonably consistent findings for higher nitrate and lower vitamin C contents of conventionally produced vegetables versus organically grown foods, particularly leafy vegetables (Williams, 2002).

Organic Food May Benefit Your Waistline

A team of European scientists found in an experiment with rats that those that ate organic food were much healthier than those that ate conventional diets. The scientists found that the organically fed rats enjoyed several health benefits, including they slept better, had stronger immune systems, and were slimmer than rats fed conventional diets (*Science Daily*, 2005).

Organic Food Allows You to Avoid Toxins

A University of Washington study analyzed pesticide breakdown products (metabolites) in pre-school aged children and found that children eating organic fruits and vegetables had concentrations of pesticide metabolites six times lower than children eating conventional produce (Curl et al, 2002).

Sustainable Agriculture

In its literal sense, sustainable agriculture refers to the ability of a farm to produce food indefinitely, without causing severe or irreversible damage to the health of the ecosystem. Two key issues are biophysical (the long-term effects of various practices on soil properties and processes essential for crop productivity) and socio-economic (the long-term ability of farmers to obtain and manage resources such as labor).

By the end of World War II, food productivity increased significantly as a result of new technologies, increased chemical use, and government subsidies. These changes allowed fewer farmers with reduced labor demands to produce the majority of the food in the United States.

Although there have been positive effects as a result of these changes, there have also been negative effects. Among these are topsoil depletion, groundwater contamination, the decline of family farms, continued neglect of the living and working conditions for farm laborers, increasing costs of production, and the disintegration of economic and social conditions in rural communities (University of California Sustainable Agriculture Research and Education Program).

The concept of sustainable agriculture addresses many environmental and social concerns, but also attempts to create viable opportunities for growers, laborers, consumers, policymakers, and many others in the entire food system. The 2008 Farm Bill, which passed on June 18, 2008, afforded significant gains in organic agriculture, conservation, and renewable energy and in securing open markets and fair contracts for livestock producers (National Campaign for Sustainable Agriculture).

Locally Grown

The local food movement is a collaborative effort to build more locally based, self-reliant food economies—one in which sustainable food production, processing, distribution, and consumption is integrated to enhance the economic, environmental, and social health of a particular place (Feenstra, 2002).

One way to support and enjoy the locally grown movement is by visiting a farmers' market. Farmers' markets allow consumers to have access to locally grown, farm-fresh produce. Additionally, farmers' markets give farmers the opportunity to develop a personal relationship with their customers and cultivate consumer loyalty. There are more than 4,600 farmers' markets operating throughout the nation today. To find a farmers' market near you, visit http://apps.ams.usda.gov/FarmersMarkets/. In addition, the National Resources Defense Council offers a state-by-state guide of foods that are in-season in any given region of the United States at http://www.nrdc.org/health/foodmiles/.

The following is a list of the produce available, by season, at the USDA Farmers' Market in Washington, DC (USDA Wholesale and Farmers' Markets).

Apples: July, August, September, October, November

Apricots: June, July, August

Asparagus: May, June

Beans: May, June, July, August, September, October

Beets: June, July, August, September, October, November

Blackberries: June, July, August, September

Blueberries: June, July, August, September

Broccoli: June, July, August, September, October

Brussels Sprouts: August, September, October

Cabbage: June, July, August, September, October, November

Cantaloupes: June, July, August

Carrots: June, July, August, September, October, November

Cherries: June, July

Corn: June, July, August, September, October

Cucumbers: June, July, August

Eggplant: June, July, August, September

Flowers: June, July, August, September, October, November

Greens: May, June, July, August, September, October, November

Grapes: July, August, September, October

Herbs: May, June, July, August, September, October, November

Leeks: September, October, November

Lettuce: May, June, July, August, September

Nectarines: July, August, September

Okra: June, July, August, September

Onions: May, June, July, August, September, October

Peaches: June, July, August, September

Pears: August, September, October, November

Peas: May, June, July

Peppers: June, July, August, September, October

Plums: July, August, September, October

Potatoes: June, July, September, October, November

Pumpkins: October, November

Radishes: May, June, July

Raspberries: June, July, August, September, October

Rhubarb: May, June, July

Squash: June, July, August, September

Strawberries: May, June, July

Tomatoes: June, July, August, September

Turnips: July, August, September

Watermelons: July, August, September

Zucchini: June, July, August, September

FUNCTIONAL FOOD

Functional food is any fresh or processed food with a claim to have a health-promoting and/or disease-preventing property beyond the basic nutritional function of supplying nutrients. Examples include fruits and vegetables, whole grains, fortified or enhanced foods and beverages, and some dietary supplements (*International Food Information Council,* 2006). The term functional food was first introduced in Japan in the mid-1980s. Japan was the first country to formulate a specific regulatory approval process for functional foods (Hasler, 1998).

The Food and Drug Administration (FDA) regulates food products according to their intended use and the nature of claims made on the package. Consumers can have peace of mind that a governmental body is regulating functional foods, although they should not automatically assume that consuming functional foods will make them healthier, cure diseases, and allow them to live longer lives. It is true, however, that enhanced foods may be useful for those with unique nutritional needs, such as vegans, who consume no animal products and need to ensure getting certain nutrients like calcium and vitamin B12. Consumers should be aware of mega-dosing on certain nutrients when consuming a lot of functional foods. For example, if you drink calcium-fortified orange juice at breakfast, take a calcium supplement, and have a latte, you may be consuming more of this particular nutrient than your body needs.

Five types of health-related statements or claims are allowed on food and dietary supplement labels:

1. *Nutrient content claims:* Indicate the presence of a specific nutrient at a certain level.
2. *Structure and function claims:* Describe the effect of dietary components on the normal structure or function of the body.

3. *Dietary guidance claims:* Describe the health benefits of broad categories of foods.

4. *Qualified health claims:* Convey a developing relationship between components in the diet and risk of disease, as reviewed by the FDA and supported by the weight of credible scientific evidence available.

5. *Health claims:* Confirm a relationship between components in the diet and risk of disease or health condition, as approved by FDA and supported by significant scientific agreement (International Food Information Council, 2006).

A large body of credible, scientific research is needed to confirm the benefits of any particular food or component. For functional foods to deliver their potential public health benefits, consumers must have a clear understanding of and a strong confidence in the scientific criteria that are used to document health statements and claims (International Food Information Council, 2006). Still, the nutritional scientific community disagree on the exact definition of a functional food.

What Are Some Functional Foods?
- Calcium-fortified orange juice
- Plant sterols: special, fortified margarines, like Promise or Benacol
- Nutrient-enhanced salad dressings with added Omega-3 Fatty Acids
- Green tea: high antioxidant levels
- Soluble fiber: oatmeal and legumes (may help lower cholesterol levels)
- Soy protein like that found in tofu (may lower cholesterol)
- Omega-3 Fatty Acids: fatty fish, added to some pastas like Barilla Plus brand, helps decrease inflammation and cholesterol levels
- Resveratrol: reduce inflammation and help reduce heart disease risk; high antioxidants, red wine/grape juice
- Lycopene: tomatoes and processed tomato products (may reduce the risk of prostate cancer), high antioxidant level
- Probiotics: fermented dairy products with live active cultures (may help support gastrointestinal health)
- Lutein: spinach, kale, collard greens (may reduce the risk of age-related macular degeneration), high antioxidant level

EATING PLANS

Several different eating plans or diets have gained significant popularity in the last decade.

The Atkins Diet Weight Loss Program

The Atkins Diet is the "father" of the high-protein, low-carbohydrate plans. Dr. Robert Atkins published his first version of the program in 1973. Today it continues to be a popular nutritional trend. The Atkins Diet advocates eliminating virtually all carbohydrates and promotes the consumption of protein. No more bagels, or pancakes at breakfast, sandwiches at lunch, or pasta at dinner. Instead, you can consume almost endless quantities of eggs, luncheon meats, beef, and poultry. The Atkins Diet is very difficult to maintain long term, but works if you think you can live the rest of your life bread-free and sugar-free, with very little fruit and a restricted list of vegetables from which to choose.

The plan is divided into four phases:

Phase 1: Induction

Phase 1 lasts a minimum of 14 days. During this phase, you must eat three regular-sized meals; eat liberal amounts of fat and protein; eat no more than 20 grams of carbohydrate per day; absolutely no fruit, bread, pasta, grains, starchy vegetables, or dairy other than cheese, cream, or butter; and avoid coffee, tea and soft drinks that contain caffeine.

Foods Allowed During Phase 1:

- Protein: chicken, turkey, lean beef, fish, shellfish, lamb, pork, veal, eggs, and a variety of vegetable proteins like tofu
- Natural fats: olive oil, safflower oil, butter, and avocado
- Leafy greens and vegetables: Salad greens and non-starchy vegetables should make up around 12 grams of carbohydrates per day
- Additional carbs daily including:

    Up to 4 ounces of cheese

    10 to 20 olives for a quick snack

    Half an avocado in a salad

    An ounce of sour cream or three ounces of unsweetened cream in coffee

    Up to 3 tablespoons lemon or lime juice

    One to two servings of Atkins bars or shakes (Check the package to see which ones are right for induction [less than 5 net carb])

Foods Not Allowed During Phase 1:

- Added sugars and trans fats though sucralose or saccharin as a sweeter is allowed. You may also have diet beverages that contain these sweeteners as well as sugar-free gelatin.
- High-carbohydrate foods including:

    Starchy vegetables such as potatoes, yams, squash

    Bread, rice, cereal and pasta

    Whole, reduced fat or skim milk

    Fruit, except for avocados, tomatoes, and olives

    Nuts or seeds

    Foods that combine protein and carbs: lentils, chickpeas (garbanzo beans), kidney beans, and other legumes

Phase 2: On-going Weight Loss (OWL)

Phase 2 is the longest phase of the Atkins Diet plan. In this phase, you steadily increase your carbohydrate consumption. Each week, you add 5 grams of carbohydrate until you eventually reach a level at which you are no longer losing weight. This is called the "Critical Carbohydrate Level for Losing." More proteins and vegetables are added, as well as berries, nuts, and seeds. If a new food causes weight gain, then you must stop eating it. This phase lasts until you have only 5 to 10 more pounds to lose. Expect to spend a few months on Phase 2 if you have more than 40 pounds to lose.

Foods Allowed During Phase 2:
- Lean protein: chicken, turkey, lean beef, fish, shellfish, lamb, pork, veal, eggs, and a variety of vegetable proteins
- Fats: olive oil, safflower oil, butter, and avocado
- Vegetables, berries, nuts, and seeds (Just remember to stick with your daily Net Carb count each week)

Phase 3: Pre-maintenance

During phase 3, you increase carbohydrate consumption until you lose less than 1 pound per week. You can add a piece of fruit or a starchy vegetable, a serving of brown rice, or sweet potatoes. Ideally, you should spend at least one month in this phase, preferably, two to three months.

Phase 4: Lifetime Maintenance

Phase 4 provides you with a way of eating so you stay slim for the rest of your life. A healthy amount of carbohydrates are allotted so you are able to maintain your weight without fluctuating more than 3 to 5 pounds.

Slim-Fast

Liquid diets have been around for a long time. Slim-Fast is well known for its "two shakes and a sensible dinner" slogan.

The Slim-Fast plan features two daily Slim-Fast meals: balanced shakes or meal bars along with a "sensible meal" and healthy snacks. This is essentially a low-fat, low-calorie, portion-controlled plan. A plus of this plan is that replacing meals with Slim-Fast products makes planning easier and can help take the guesswork out of food selection.

Dieters using this plan must buy a lot of the Slim-Fast products, which can be costly. In addition, the long-term use of the Slim-Fast products may become unrealistic. Obviously, a person has to like the way the products taste, or they will not stick to the plan.

The ingredients lists of many of the Slim-Fast products are quite long and highly processed. A whole foods based diet would be preferable. It is best to save your money and learn to eat right without trendy and highly processed, expensive, packaged products.

Weight Watchers

Weight Watchers has been around since the 1960s and recognizes dieting as just one part of long-term weight management. The Weight Watchers philosophy promotes results from a healthy lifestyle, which encompasses all aspects: mental, emotional, and physical health.

Weight Watchers does not specify what you may or may not eat. The goal of Weight Watchers is to help people make healthy eating decisions and encourage them to enjoy more physical activity, thereby losing weight safely and sensibly and, most importantly, keeping it off.

The Weight Watchers program allows you to choose from one of two plans based on good, old-fashioned "calories in, calories out" advice.

The Flex Plan

This flex plan promotes the original Weight Watchers philosophy: "Eat the food you love and lose weight." No foods are prohibited; instead, each food is assigned points based on the food's calorie, total fat, and dietary fiber content.

This system guides food choices by encouraging a selection of healthy foods. Some examples are:

1 cup broccoli = 0 points

½ cantaloupe = 2 points

1 small bean burrito = 5 points

1 cup spaghetti with ½ cup marinara sauce = 6 points

1 6-ounce steak = 8 points

1 3-ounce grilled chicken breast = 3 points

¼ cup regular creamy salad dressing = 8 points

1 slice bread = 2 points

1 ounce chocolate = 4 points

1 scoop vanilla ice cream = 4 points

Each person has a target daily points range, calculated based on his or her body weight. For example, a 5-foot-6-inch woman who weighs 180 pounds would be allotted between 22 and 27 points each day. A "points finder" helps members calibrate the points value of a recipe or a packaged product using the nutrition facts label.

The initial Weight Watchers' goal is to reduce body weight by 5 percent to 10 percent, and the ultimate weight goal is a body mass index less than 25. For those who have a lot of weight to lose, the goal is to lose in increments of 10 percent, which helps people stay motivated.

The Core Plan

The core plan is a newer approach for Weight Watchers that allows members to control calories by focusing their eating on a core list of wholesome nutritious foods, but without counting or tracking. The list includes foods from all the food groups: fruits and vegetables; grains and starches; lean meats, fish, and poultry; eggs, and dairy products. The foods in this core list are low in fat and calories. An occasional treat outside the list is allowed.

The Zone Diet

The Zone Diet is a diet popularized by biochemist Barry Sears. It advocates consuming calories from carbohydrates, protein and fat in a 40:30:30 ratio.

"The Zone" is Sears' name for proper hormone balance. He argues that when insulin levels are neither too high nor too low, and glucagon levels are not too high, specific anti-inflammatory chemicals are released. The diet claims that a 30:40 ratio of protein to carbohydrates triggers this effect, and this is called "The Zone." Sears claims that these natural anti-inflammatories are heart and health-friendly. This "hormonally correct diet" claims lasting fat loss, greater health, and peak athletic, mental, and emotional performance, as well as a longer lifespan.

The cardinal rule of the Zone Diet is to ensure that each meal and snack has the right combination of low-fat protein, "good" carbs, and a bit of fat. Meal timing is also essential to ensure adequate "medication" every four to six hours.

Ultimately, the Zone Diet is easier than the Atkins Diet in terms of restriction and maintenance. Still, some who follow the diet report feeling fatigued and find it hard to maintain.

ASSIGNMENT #6

Name: _____

Date: _____

1. Have you ever followed one of the eating plans discussed in the chapter? Describe how you felt while doing it. If not, do you know anyone who has followed one of these eating plans? How did it work for him or her?

_____
_____
_____
_____
_____
_____
_____
_____
_____
_____
_____
_____
_____
_____
_____
_____
_____

2. Do you buy organic foods? Why or why not?

_____
_____
_____
_____
_____
_____
_____
_____
_____
_____
_____
_____

3. Have you ever shopped at a farmers' market? What did you buy? If not, would you shop at one? Why or why not?

_____
_____
_____
_____
_____
_____
_____
_____
_____
_____
_____
_____
_____
_____
_____
_____

4. Do you eat any functional foods? If so, which ones? After learning about functional foods, do you think you will include them in your daily diet? Why or why not?

_____
_____
_____
_____
_____
_____
_____
_____
_____
_____
_____
_____
_____
_____
_____
_____

RESOURCES

Curl, C. L., Fenske, R. A., Elgethun, K. (2002). Organophosphorus pesticide exposure on urban and suburban pre-school children with organic and conventional diets. *Environmental Health Perspectives,* National Institute of Environmental Sciences.

Feenstra, G. (2002). Creating space for sustainable food systems: lessons from the field. *Agriculture and Human Values* 19(2): 99–106.

Hansen, N. (2004). Organic food sales see healthy growth. MSNBC.com, retrieved on October 20, 2008.

Hasler, C. M. (1998). Functional foods: Their role in disease prevention and health promotion. *Food Technology* 52(2):57–62.

International Food Information Council (November, 2006). http://www.ific.org/nutrition/functional/index.cfm, retrieved on October 27, 2008.

National Campaign for Sustainable Agriculture. http://www.sustainableagriculture.net/site/PageServer?pagename=About_Main, retrieved on October 20, 2008.

National Resources Defense Council: Eat Local. http://www.nrdc.org/health/foodmiles/, retrieved October 20, 2008.

Organic Food Standards and Labels: The Facts. National Organic Program. Retrieved on October 20, 2008.

United States Department of Agriculture National Organic Program: Labeling Packaged Products, January 9, 2003.

United States Department Agriculture Wholesale and Farmers Markets. http://www.ams.usda.gov/AMSv1.0/ams.fetchTemplateData.do?template=TemplateN&navID=WFMUSDAMarketSeasonalProduce&rightNav1=WFMUSDAMarketSeasonalProduce&topNav=&leftNav=WholesaleandFarmersMarkets&page=WFMUSDAMarketSeasonalProduce&resultType=&acct=frmrdir, retrieved October 20, 2008.

University of California Sustainable Agriculture Research and Education Program. http://www.sarep.ucdavis.edu/Concept.htm, retrieved on October 20, 2008.

University of Newcastle Upon Tyne (2005, March 29). Organic Diet Makes Rats Healthier. *ScienceDaily.* Retrieved October 20, 2008, from http://www.sciencedaily.com-/releases/2005/03/050328182123.htm.

Williams, C. M. (2002). Nutritional quality of organic food: Shades of grey or shades of green? *Proceedings of the Nutrition Society* 61:19–24.

DANGERS IN OUR FOOD SUPPLY

Hazards in food cause an estimated 76 million illnesses, 325,000 hospitalizations, and 5,000 deaths in the United States each year, most of which are never reported to public health officials. These illnesses cost American taxpayers approximately $6.9 billion annually in medical costs, hospitalizations, and lost work time, according to the United States Department of Agriculture (USDA). Despite advances in food production and processing, foodborne illnesses from hazards such as Salmonella, E. coli O157:H7, and Listeria, continue to be a significant public health problem. At greatest risk are older Americans, children, pregnant women and their unborn children, and those with compromised immune systems.

Across spectrums of gender, race, age and socio-economic status, Americans are sicker than people in other western countries. This is in large part due to the adulteration of our food supply. In the United States, more than 3,000 substances can be added to foods for the purpose of preservation, coloring, texture, increasing flavor and more. Although each of these substances is legal to use (at least in the United States), whether or not they are all something you want to be consuming is another story altogether.

INGREDIENTS TO AVOID

The first step to start a healthier lifestyle is to pay attention to the ingredients in the foods you buy. If you cannot pronounce the ingredients, chances are you should not be eating them. Healthy foods should contain simple ingredients that are easily recognizable. You should also be careful about purchasing an item that has more than five to seven ingredients in it.

A simple general rule is to avoid as many additives as possible, especially:

- Partially hydrogenated fats
- High fructose corn syrup
- Sodium nitrite and/or nitrates
- Fake sugars
- Olestra
- Monosodium glutamate (MSG)
- Acesulfame K
- Excessive salt and sugar
- Artificial coloring

Monosodium Glutamate (MSG)

MSG is used as a flavor enhancer in many packaged foods, including soups, salad dressings, sausages, hot dogs, canned tuna, potato chips, and many more. Many consumers have experienced the ill effects of MSG, which leave them with a headache, nausea, or vomiting after eating MSG-containing foods. MSG is known as an excitotoxin which is a group of excitatory amino acids that can cause sensitive neurons to die.

According to the FDA, MSG Symptom Complex Can Result in:
- Numbness
- Burning sensation
- Tingling
- Facial pressure or tightness
- Chest pain
- Headache
- Nausea
- Rapid heartbeat
- Drowsiness
- Weakness
- Difficulty breathing for asthmatics

Americans associate MSG with Chinese food; however, MSG is in many more foods than Chinese food, and is listed under many other names than MSG. Some ingredient labels hide MSG under names that consumers won't recognize, such as hydrolyzed soy protein. In terms of labeling requirements, the FDA says that "monosodium glutamate" must be listed on the label only if MSG is added to a food. However, it's misleading for a manufacturer to list "No MSG," or "No Added MSG" on foods if sources of free glutamates, like hydrolyzed protein, exist. Further, items listed as "flavors," "natural flavors," or "flavorings" may not include MSG, hydrolyzed proteins, or autolyzed yeast.

MSG Is Found in:
- Autolyzed yeast
- Calcium caseinate
- Gelatin
- Glutamate
- Glutamic acid
- Hydrolyzed protein
- Monopotassium glutamate
- Monosodium glutamate
- Sodium caseinate
- Textured protein
- Yeast extract
- Yeast food
- Yeast nutrient

High Fructose Corn Syrup

The process for making the sweetener high fructose corn syrup (HFCS) out of corn was developed in the 1970s. Until the 1970s most of the sugar we ate came from sucrose derived from sugar beets or sugar cane. Then sugar from corn-corn syrup, fructose, dextrose, dextrine, and especially high fructose corn syrup (HFCS) began to gain popularity as a sweetener because it was much less expensive to produce. High fructose corn syrup can be manipulated to contain equal amounts of fructose and glucose, or up to 80 percent fructose and 20 percent glucose. Thus, with almost twice the fructose, HFCS delivers a double danger compared to sugar. Today Americans consume more HFCS than sugar. HCFS is produced by processing corn starch to yield glucose, and then processing the glucose to produce a high percentage of fructose.

Consumers may think that because it contains fructose, which they associate with fruit, that it is healthier than sugar. A team of investigators at the USDA have discovered that this isn't so.

Sucrose is composed of glucose and fructose. When sugar is given to rats in high amounts, the rats develop multiple health problems, especially when the rats were deficient in certain nutrients, such as copper. The researchers wanted to know whether it was the fructose or the glucose that was causing the problems, so they repeated their studies with two groups of rats, one given high amounts of glucose and one given high amounts of fructose. The glucose group was unaffected, but the fructose group had disastrous results. The male rats did not reach adulthood. They had anemia, high cholesterol, and heart hypertrophy (hearts enlarged until they exploded). They also had delayed testicular development. All fructose must be metabolized in the liver.

The livers of the rats on the high fructose diet looked like the livers of alcoholics, plugged with fat and cirrhotic. Because it is metabolized by the liver, fructose does not cause the pancreas to release insulin the way it normally does. Fructose converts to fat more than any other sugar. Fructose also raises serum triglycerides significantly. This may be one of the reasons Americans continue to get fatter.

Aspartame (Equal, NutraSweet)

Aspartame is the artificial sweetener found in Equal and NutraSweet, along with products that contain them (diet sodas and other low-calorie and diet foods). This sweetener has been found to cause brain tumors in rats as far back as the 1970s; however, recent studies have found that even small doses increase the incidence of lymphomas and leukemia in rats, along with brain tumors. People who are sensitive to aspartame may also suffer from headaches, dizziness, and hallucinations after consuming it.

Acesulfame-K

Acesulfame-K is an artificial sweetener that is about 200 times sweeter than sugar. It's used in baked goods, chewing gum, gelatin desserts, and soft drinks. Two rat studies have found that this substance may cause cancer. Acesulfame-K also breaks down into acetoacetamide, which has been found to affect the thyroid in rats, rabbits, and dogs.

Olestra

Olestra is a fat substitute used in crackers and potato chips, marketed under the brand name Olean. This synthetic fat is not absorbed by the body, (instead it goes right through it) causing diarrhea, loose stools, abdominal cramps and flatulence. Furthermore, olestra reduces the body's ability to absorb beneficial fat-soluble nutrients, including lycopene, lutein, and beta-carotene.

Sodium Nitrite (Sodium Nitrate)

Sodium nitrite (or sodium nitrate) is used as a preservative, coloring, and flavoring in bacon, ham, hot dogs, luncheon meats, corned beef, smoked fish, and other processed meats. These additives can lead to the formation of cancer-causing chemicals called nitrosamines. Some studies have found a link between consuming cured meats and nitrite and cancer in humans.

Hydrogenated Vegetable Oil (Trans Fat)

An artificial ingredient in foods, trans fat is made when manufacturers add hydrogen to vegetable oil in an effort to increase the shelf life and flavor stability of foods containing these fats. This promotes heart disease and diabetes. Trans fats are believed to be harmful because they contribute to heart disease by raising bad cholesterol and lowering good cholesterol at the same time. The Institute of Medicine has advised that consumers should eat as little trans fat as possible. You should avoid anything with these ingredients on the label, which includes some margarine, vegetable shortening, crackers, cookies, baked goods, salad dressings, bread, and more. New York is the nation's first city to ban artery-clogging artificial trans fats in all its restaurants and other food service establishments.

Blue 1 and Blue 2

Blue 1, which is used to color candy, beverages and baked goods, may cause cancer. Blue 2, found in pet food, candy and beverages, has caused brain tumors in mice.

Red 3

Red 3 is a food coloring used in cherries (in fruit cocktails), baked goods, and candy. It causes thyroid tumors in rats, and may cause them in humans as well.

Yellow 6

As the third most often used food coloring, yellow 6 is found in many products, including baked goods, candy, gelatin and sausages. Yellow 6 has been found to cause adrenal gland and kidney tumors, and contains small amounts of many carcinogens.

HOW CLEAN IS OUR WATER?

Roughly 70 percent of the earth's surface is covered in water. Even though water seems to be everywhere, not all of it is suitable for use as drinking water. Of all the water on earth, only 3 percent is fresh water, with much of it frozen or underground. Less than one percent of the water on earth can be used as drinking water. Before we drink it and before it is released back into surface waters (such as rivers and lakes), our water must go through a variety of treatment processes.

Drinking water comes from a variety of sources. Some of the water comes from water purification plants. Some comes from underground sources. Due to the diversity of the sources, the water that we drink can differ greatly in quality and healthiness. In many instances, you cannot tell if water is contaminated by taste, smell, or by how it looks. Many common pesticides, herbicides, chemicals, and cleaners are leached into our water supply.

Bottled vs. Tap Water

Bottled water is a booming industry that grosses more than $7 billion dollars a year in the United States. Up to 40 percent of bottled water is bottled tap water that may or may not have received additional treatment. The Environmental Protection Agency (EPA) regulates the quality of public water supplies; however, it has no authority over bottled water. Further, bottled water labels can be misleading and may depict mountains and streams when the water actually came from a well in an industrial facility parking lot.

Too many factors beyond our control can drastically impact our tap water quality. Pollution in the form of chemical spills, leaking fuel tanks, pesticides, cleaning fluids, weed killers, and fertilizers is just the tip of the water-contamination iceberg. Even the very chemicals that water companies add to our water to "protect" us like fluoride, chlorine, and other disinfectants can lead to health risks.

The **Safe Drinking Water Act** requires that all drinking water go through a treatment process before it is sent to our taps.

Local water suppliers that use water from a local surface water (rivers, lakes, or reservoirs) must use a treatment process to take out any dirt particles, other organic matter (such as leaves and sticks), and contaminants. The suppliers add chemicals called coagulants so that this matter will form clumps and settle to the bottom of the tanks that store the water. Once the clumps settle, the water is put through a filter to remove any microscopic germs.

Water suppliers that use water from an underground source use a different process. Ground water is naturally filtered as it passes through the earth into underground reservoirs called aquifers. Water that comes from wells usually does not contain as much organic material as water from rivers and reservoirs.

The most common drinking water treatment is disinfection. Most water suppliers add chlorine or other disinfectants to kill bacteria and other germs. They may use other treatments to make the water clean and safe, depending on the quality of their source water. Bottled water, on the other hand, utilizes ozone disinfection, which is tasteless and odorless.

According to a survey of 42 states by the nonprofit Environmental Working Group, a research organization in Washington, D.C., water supplies across the country meet current standards set by the U.S. Environmental Protection Agency, but contain 141 chemicals that are not regulated by the agency.

Go to www.ewg.org/tapwater/yourwater/index.php, or contact your local water supplier and request a quality report, which will usually detail where your water comes from and exactly what is in it. Environmental groups have also voiced concerns over the huge amounts of waste and toxins created by the bottled water industry.

One of the most overlooked sources of water contamination is water pipes. The EPA reported that even safe, potable water often becomes contaminated after it leaves the municipal treatment plant. The EPA said that sediment, such as scales and microbial material (or "biofilm"), builds up inside pipe walls and leaches into the drinking water as it passes through on the way to your home. If the water's pH is low, the acidity can result in materials like iron, copper, lead, zinc, arsenic and manganese showing up at levels well beyond state and federal drinking water standards.

In any given year, about 25 percent of beaches in the United States are under advisories or are closed at least one time because of contamination with pathogenic bacteria, viruses, or parasites. Each year, plastic waste in water and coastal areas kills up to 100,000 marine mammals, one million sea birds, and countless fish. Around 80 percent of the pollution in seas and oceans comes from land-based activities. Water pollution is caused primarily by the drainage of contaminated waters into surface water or groundwater.

Pesticides and herbicides contain toxic materials that pose both environmental and human health risks. More than 14 million Americans drink water contaminated with pesticides, and the EPA estimates that 10 percent of wells contain pesticides.

Municipal water pollution consists of waste water from homes and commercial establishments. Drain and oven cleaners, paint thinners, and bathroom cleaners are just a few of the items we use that can cause serious health and environmental problems.

Is Bottled Water Safer?

A study by the Natural Resources Defense Council, an environmental action group, found that bottled water is no safer than tap water on average, and is sometimes less safe, containing elevated levels of arsenic, bacteria, and other contaminants. Some environmentalists, shareholder activists, and church groups are targeting Coca-Cola, PepsiCo, and Nestle, the leading sellers of bottled water. Some examples include:

- The Natural Resources Defense Council, Sierra Club and World Wildlife Federation have all urged their supporters to consume less bottled water. A 1999 NRDC study found that bottled water was no purer or safer than most tap water.
- A handful of high-end restaurants have stopped serving bottled water.

Pepsi's Aquafina, the best-selling brand, and Coke's Dasani, which is second, are made from purified tap water. In fact, the Sierra Club states that Coca Cola's Dasani and Pepsi's Aquafina are tap water coming from places like Queens, New York and Jacksonville, Florida with some additional treatment. Nestle, the global leader, gets most of its water from spring sources; they are sold in North America under such regional brands as Ice Mountain, Deer Park, Poland Spring, Arrowhead, Ozarka, Zephyrhills, and Calistoga.

The Food and Drug Administration has established "Standards of Identity" for bottled water sold in the United States. Here are some of the more common identities:

Artesian water—originates from a confined aquifer that has been tapped and in which the water level stands at some height above the top of the aquifer.

Fluoridated water—contains fluoride added within the limitations established in the FDA Code of Federal Regulations.

Ground water—is from an underground source that is under a pressure equal to or greater than atmospheric pressure.

Purified water—has been produced by distillation, deionization, reverse osmosis, or other suitable processes. Purified water may also be referred to as "demineralized water."

Spring water—comes from an underground formation from which water flows naturally to the Earth's surface.

Well water—is taken from a hole tapping. This hole may be bored, drilled, or otherwise constructed in the ground.

Mineral water is drawn from an underground source and contains at least 250 ppm of dissolved salts. Whichever minerals are present are what make mineral water what it is. Some minerals that may appear in mineral water include calcium, iron, and sodium.

Sparkling water is carbonated (contains CO_2, producing the "fizz"). It can either be naturally carbonated or mechanically carbonated in a process where CO_2 is added to normal tap water.

Seltzer water is tap water that has been filtered and carbonated. Club soda is seltzer water with added mineral salts.

Sterilized water is used to make baby formula and is also drunk by people with immuno-compromised systems. It must be processed to meet FDA's requirements for commercial sterility.

Distilled or de-mineralized water is usually tap water that has been treated to remove nearly all minerals and sodium that occur naturally in water. Since distilled water is like a vacuum without any minerals, it will actually leach beneficial minerals from your body to balance it out.

How Can I Make My Water Safe?

Everyday household activities are a major contributor to polluted runoff, which is among the most serious sources of water contamination. When it rains, fertilizer from lawns, oil from driveways, paint, and solvent residues from walls and decks, and even waste from pets are all washed into storm sewers or nearby lakes, rivers, and streams—the same lakes, rivers, and streams that we rely on for drinking, bathing, swimming, and fishing.

- Don't drink water straight from lakes, rivers, streams, or springs.
- Because you cannot be sure if your tap water is safe, you may wish to avoid tap water, including water or ice from a refrigerator ice-maker, which is made with tap water.
- You may also wish to boil or filter your water.
- Boiling is the best way to kill germs in your water.
- Heat your water at a rolling boil for 1 minute.
- After the boiled water cools, put it in a clean bottle or pitcher with a lid and store it in the refrigerator.
- Use the water for drinking, cooking, or making ice.
- Water bottles and ice trays should be cleaned with soap and water before use.

Environmental Impact

Fossil Fuel Consumption

Approximately 1.5 million gallons of oil—enough to run 100,000 cars for a whole year—are used to make plastic water bottles, and transporting these bottles burns thousands more gallons of oil. In addition, the burning of the oil and other fossil fuels, which also are used to generate the energy that powers the manufacturing process, emits global warming pollution into the atmosphere.

Waste

Only about 10 percent of plastic water bottles are recycled, leaving the rest in landfills where it takes thousands of years for the materials to decompose.

Water Bottles

Over the past decade, evidence has been building that a variety of pesticides, plastics, and solvents containing chemicals can alter normal development in both wild and domestic animals.

Look at the triangle (▲) symbol underneath your water bottle and you will see a number inside the triangle. Polycarbonate water bottles (labeled #7) contain bisphenol A (BPA), which leaches from the plastic even at room temperature and has been linked to chromosome damage and hormone disruption. The chemical in question, Bisphenol A (BPA), has been linked to breast and uterine cancer, as well as decreased testosterone levels. These are the types of plastic Nalgene water bottles found in sports stores. #1 PET or PETE bottles (polyethylene terephthalate) may leach DEHA, a known carcinogen, if used more than once. Additionally, your water bottle that has been refilled is likely to contain potentially harmful bacteria that grow on saliva, food particles, and fecal material from unwashed hands. Many people have reported getting diarrhea from their reused water bottles. Washing bottles with hot water and detergent or a rinse with bleach will sanitize them, but also leaches harmful chemicals out of the plastic.

What to Do?

Use metal bottles. A Swiss company, SIGG, makes colorful and safe aluminum drinking bottles lined with an impermeable alloy. They can be found on the Internet.

Relatively Safe Plastics
- #1 polyethylene terephalate (PET) used only *once*
- #2 and #4 polyethylene
- # 5 polypropylene (catsup bottles, yogurt containers)

Unsafe Plastics

- **#3 V (Vinyl) or PVC** is found in cooking oil bottles and clear food packaging.

  Number 3 plastics may release toxic breakdown products (including pthalates) into food and drinks. The risk is highest when containers start wearing out, are put through the dishwasher, or when they are heated (including microwaves). PVC manufacturing can release highly toxic dioxins into the environment, and the materials can off-gas toxic plasticizers into your home.

- **#6 polystyrene (Styrofoam)** is found in disposable plates and cups, meat trays, egg cartons, and carry-out containers.

  Number 6 plastics can release potentially toxic breakdown products (including styrene), particularly when heated, including that insulated coffee cup.

- **#7 polycarbonate (Nalgene)** is found in baby bottles, three- and five-gallon water bottles, and certain food containers.

  A wide range of plastic resins that don't fit into the other six categories are lumped into number 7. Some are quite safe, but the ones to worry about are the hard polycarbonate varieties, as found in various drinking containers (like Nalgene bottles) and rigid plastic baby bottles. Studies have shown polycarbonate can leach bisphenol A, a potential hormone disruptor, into liquids.

Never Use:

- Food or drinks heated in plastic containers in a microwave.
- Styrofoam cups (polystyrene #6), especially for hot liquids.
- #7 polycarbonate (Nalgene) water bottles
- Plastic baby bottles. If you must use bottles, use only glass baby bottles with silicone, not latex, nipples.
- Do not reuse plastic water bottles.

HOW SAFE IS AMERICA'S MEAT AND FISH SUPPLY?

The Centers for Disease Control and Prevention estimates that food-borne hazards are the cause of 76 million cases of illness each year, including 325,000 hospitalizations. Two million of those reports are caused by bacteria commonly found in meat.

In *The Jungle,* Upton Sinclair described slaughterhouse conditions and meat contamination so horrific that the government stepped in and created a new agency to monitor the business: the Food and Drug Administration (FDA). The public's response to this book prompted the government to pass the Meat Inspection Act in 1906. The act empowered the U.S. Department of Agriculture (USDA) to require sanitary equipment, conditions, and methods, and to ban the use of harmful chemicals and preservatives in slaughtering and packing plants. Unfortunately the story did not end happily ever after.

In 2007, there were more than 20 beef recalls in the United States, totaling 33.4 million pounds. Most were prompted by the public health threat of harmful bacteria, such as *E. coli* and *salmonella.* In February 2008, a YouTube video showed disturbing images of sick cows in a meat processing plant in California. The video showed how "downer cows"—those so injured or sick that they can't stand up—were processed and entered into the nation's food supply. Particularly troubling is that about a quarter of the recalled meat, which amounts to about 37 million pounds, went to schools and federal nutrition programs in 36 states.

Watch video at: www.youtube.com/watch?v=vcvBG4FWPDg.

Food safety groups have voiced criticism over these numbers, saying that there are too few eye-balls watching too much meat. The USDA is underfunded and understaffed. A second question among food safety advocates is whether the USDA is doing enough to make sure that plants have adequate safety plans in place. Currently, the USDA employs 7,500 inspectors for 6,300 federal plants (the majority of which are slaughterhouses) which is roughly one inspector per plant, although in practice teams of inspectors tend to cover multiple plants. The USDA is also currently operating with an overall vacancy rate of 9 percent for inspectors.

Agricultural Practices

Some chickens never see a barnyard but instead spend their short lives in a windowless warehouse where every aspect of the birds' environment is controlled to make them grow as quickly and inexpensively as possible. It is not uncommon to have as many as 80,000 birds per warehouse. This is too large a flock to create any sense of social (or pecking) order among the chickens, so they go crazy pecking each other, sometimes to death. It is also a common practice to debeak the birds to make life easier in the crowded warehouse.

These birds grow so fast and so fat that many develop skeletal disorders that prevent them from walking or standing. Their life span averages only about two months instead of an expected 15 to 20 years for a free-roaming chicken. Because their laboratory feed is loaded with antibiotics, sulfa drugs, arsenic compounds, growth hormones, and pesticides, these birds are not exactly a picture of health. Dietary deficiencies can result in retarded growth, deformities, blindness, and disease.

A cow's life on the farm is equally "glamorous." After birth, most bulls are castrated and dehorned. Cattle are then allowed to roam on the range for six months to a year until they are sent off to a standing-room-only feedlot where they are fattened up for slaughter. To obtain the optimum weight in the least amount of time, feedlot managers implant time-release anabolic steroid pellets in the cattle's ears, which will increase their hormone levels two to five times. Routine use of human antibiotics in animal production may produce resistant strains of bacteria which can be transferred to humans. Besides growth hormones and antibiotics, pesticide and herbicide residues are another potential danger to the meat eaters of America.

The Slaughterhouse

Even healthy farm animals raised in a clean environment can become contaminated during processing and packing. Working conditions in a slaughterhouse are far from ideal. Low-paid workers suffer a high rate of personal injury and disability, the second highest of any occupation in the United States. Up to half of the poultry workers suffer from repetitive motion syndrome, such as carpal tunnel, due to the fast pace and high volume. Sixty to seventy chickens may be checked by one person per hour. Workers are cutting up to 300 cows an hour, working long hours with few breaks. Many plants have an employee turnover rate of more than 40 percent, resulting in too many untrained workers. Because union membership is discouraged and workers are worried about job security, nothing is done to remedy dangerous working environments.

Mercury

Mercury occurs naturally in the environment and can also be released into the air through industrial pollution. Mercury falls from the air and can accumulate in streams and oceans which is turned into methylmercury in the water. Fish absorb the methylmercury as they feed in these waters and, as a result, it accumulates in their tissues. In America 1 in 6 children born every year has been exposed to mercury levels so high that he or she is potentially at risk for learning disabilities, motor skill impairment, and short-term memory loss.

Fish and shellfish are an important part of a healthy diet. Fish and shellfish contain high-quality protein and other essential nutrients, are low in saturated fat, and contain omega-3 fatty acids. A well-balanced diet that includes a variety of fish and shellfish can contribute to heart health; however, some fish and shellfish contain higher levels of mercury that may harm an unborn baby or young child's developing nervous system. The risks from mercury in fish and shellfish depend on the quantity and types of seafood consumed. The Food and Drug Administration (FDA) and the Environmental Protection Agency (EPA) advise women who may become pregnant, pregnant women, nursing mothers, and young children to avoid some types of fish and eat fish and shellfish that are lower in mercury.

1. Avoid shark, swordfish, king mackerel, and tilefish because they contain high levels of mercury.
2. Eat up to 12 ounces (2 average meals) a week of a variety of fish and shellfish that are lower in mercury.
   - Five of the most commonly eaten fish that are low in mercury are shrimp, canned light tuna, wild salmon, pollock, and catfish.
3. Do not eat "farm raised" fish. Farm raised means that they are raised in pens, don't get lots of swimming room, are fed pellets that have been shown to be contaminated, are prone to disease (and therefore fed antibiotics) and can get out and infect the fish in the wild. They are also highest in mercury.

To review a list of fish to consume or avoid, visit: http://www.mbayaq.org/cr/cr_seafoodwatch/download.asp.

Best Choices

Arctic char (farmed)

Barramundi (U.S. farmed)

Catfish (U.S. farmed)

Clams, mussels, oysters (farmed)

Clams: softshell/steamers (wild)

Crab: Dungeness

Croaker: Atlantic

Halibut: Pacific

Herring: Atlantic/sardines

Lobster: Spiny (U.S.)

Pollock (Alaska wild)

Salmon (Alaska wild)

Scallops: Bay (farmed)

Squid: Longfin (U.S.)

Striped bass (farmed or wild)

Sturgeon, caviar (farmed)

Swordfish (Canada, U.S. harpoon, handline)

Tilapia (U.S. farmed)

Trout: Rainbow (farmed)

Tuna: Albacore (U.S., British Columbia troll/polc)

Tuna: Skipjack (troll/pole)

Good Alternatives

Basa, swai (farmed)

Black sea bass

Bluefish

Clams: Atlantic surf, hard, ocean

Quahog (wild)

Crab: Blue, Jonah, King (U.S.), Snow

Crab: Imitation/surimi

Haddock (hook and line)

Hake: Silver, red and offshore

Lobster: American/Maine

Mahi mahi/dolphinfish (U.S.)

Oysters (wild)

Scallops: Sea (Canada and Northeast)

Scup/porgy

Shrimp: Northern

Shrimp (U.S. farmed or wild)

Squid

Swordfish (U.S. longline)

Tilefish (Mid-Atlantic)

Tuna: Bigeye, yellowfin (troll/pole)

Tuna: canned light, canned-white/albacore

Avoid

Chilean seabass/toothfish

Cod: Atlantic

Crab: King (imported)

Dogfish (Atlantic)

Flounders, soles (Atlantic)

Haddock (trawled)

Hake: White

Halibut: Atlantic

Mahi mahi/dolphinfish (imported)

Monkfish

Orange roughy

Salmon (farmed, including Atlantic)

Scallops: Sea (Mid-Atlantic)

Sharks and skates

Shrimp (imported farmed or wild)

Snapper: Red

Sturgeon, caviar (imported wild)

Swordfish (imported)

Tilefish (Southeast)

Tuna: Albacore, bigeye, yellowfin

Tuna: Bluefin

Source: www.oceansalive.org/eat.cfm

What Can We Do?

If we choose to include meat in our diet, then how can we ensure that we are eating the safest food possible? Raising our own chickens or becoming vegetarians may be excellent alternatives. If that is not an option, consider buying naturally raised or organic meat and poultry. USDA ratings such as "prime" and "choice" refer to the marbling or fat content of the meat, not the quality. If you can't find naturally raised poultry or your grocer will not order it, look for kosher poultry, which is processed and handled according to kosher requirements.

Kosher laws are stricter than USDA standards, when it comes to the health of animals that can be eaten. They prohibit, for example, using cows with broken bones or animals that are visibly sick. The laws strictly dictate how the animals are fed, killed and processed. Like organic meat and poultry, kosher meats and poultry are hormone free.

The USDA approved four categories of organic labels, based on the percentage of organic content.

1. **100 Percent Organic** may carry the USDA Organic Seal.
2. **Organic** requires at least 95 percent of content to be organic by weight (excluding water and salt) to carry the USDA Organic Seal.
3. **Made with Organic** requires at least 70 percent of content to be organic and the front product panel to display the phrase "Made with Organic," followed by up to three specific ingredients (may not display the new USDA Organic seal.)
4. **Less than 70% of content is organic** may list only those ingredients that are organic on the ingredient panel with no mention of organic on the main panel (may not display the new USDA Organic seal)

Reading the stickers found on produce is an easy way to find organic fruits and vegetables. A 5-digit number beginning with 9 means it was grown organically. A 4-digit number means the food was conventionally grown. For example, the sticker on an organic apple would read "93012." A conventional one would say "4011." (Organic Trade Association)

Be careful not to cross-contaminate by spreading raw meat juices onto knives and cutting boards. Most bacteria, unlike chemical residues, will die when cooked thoroughly so forget about those medium-rare burgers on the grill (the grill and the microwave both cook unevenly). Ground meat is especially high risk because it can be a combination of around-the-world beef or old beef mixed with fresher beef.

Reducing Risk

The EPA offers the following suggestions:

• Wash and scrub all fresh fruits and vegetables under running water or using a vegetable wash.
• Peel fruits and vegetables when possible
• Discard the outer leaves of leafy vegetables
• Trim fat from meat and skin from poultry. Pesticide residue can collect in fat.
• Eating a variety of foods from a variety of sources will reduce the likelihood of repeated exposure to a single pesticide.

The Environmental Working Group has created this ranking of produce by pesticide residue to help you make better choices.

The Full List: 43 Fruits and Vegetables

Rank	Fruit and Vegetable	Score
1 (worst)	Peaches	100 (highest pesticide load)
2	Apples	96
3	Sweet bell peppers	86
4	Celery	85
5	Nectarines	84
6	Strawberries	83
7	Cherries	75
8	Lettuce	69
9	Grapes (imported)	68
10	Pears	65
11	Spinach	60
12	Potatoes	58
13	Carrots	57
14	Green beans	55
15	Hot peppers	53
16	Cucumbers	52
17	Raspberries	47
18	Plums	46
19	Oranges	46
20	Grapes domestic	46
21	Cauliflower	39
22	Tangerine	38
23	Mushrooms	37
24	Cantaloupe	34
25	Lemon	31
26	Honeydew melon	31
27	Grapefruit	31
28	Winter squash	31
29	Tomatoes	30
30	Sweet potatoes	30
31	Watermelon	25
32	Blueberries	24
33	Papaya	21
34	Eggplant	19
35	Broccoli	18
36	Cabbage	17
37	Bananas	16
38	Kiwi	14
39	Asparagus	11
40	Sweet peas frozen	11
41	Mango	9
42	Pineapples	7
43	Sweet corn frozen	2
44	Avocado	1
45 (best)	Onions	1 (lowest pesticide load)

Courtesy of the Environmental Working Group, Washington, D.C.

FOODBORNE ILLNESS

A foodborne illness is a disease carried or transmitted to people by food. Food poisoning, on the other hand, refers to the actual point in time when a food is contaminated. Each year, millions of people are affected by foodborne illness, although the majority of cases are not reported. In fact, the Centers for Disease Control (CDC) estimates 76 million cases of foodborne illness occur yearly in the United States. Among the more serious cases each year, 325,000 require hospitalization and 5,000 result in death. (www.cdc.gov)

Am I At Risk for Foodborne Illness?

Anyone who eats food is theoretically at risk of developing foodborne illness. However, there are certain populations, also known as *high-risk populations,* who have a higher risk of contracting a foodborne illness than others, sometimes with serious results.

They include:

- *Infants and preschool-age children:* Young children are at a higher risk because they have not yet built adequate immune systems.
- *Elderly people:* Almost opposite of young children, older folks' immunity is on the decline and weakening with age. Also, their sense of taste and smell is not as strong.
- *Pregnant women:* A pregnant woman is at higher risk for foodborne illness and should avoid certain foods such as: deli meats, soft cheese, shellfish, raw sprouts, or undercooked meats and poultry.
- *People taking certain medications:* Ingesting certain medications such as immunosuppressants (for diseases such as HIV/AIDS, cancer, lupus, etc.) and antibiotics increase susceptibility to pathogens present on food.
- *People with chronic illness:* Anyone who has just had major surgery, who is an organ donor/recipient, or those with illnesses like diabetes have a higher likelihood of contracting a foodborne illness.

Because these groups are of particular concern for contracting foodborne illness, it is especially important that they eat foods that are kept cold and are cooked to the appropriate internal temperature.

Riskiest Foods

When thinking of foods likely to cause foodborne illness, what comes to mind for most people are foods and condiments such as mayonnaise or ground beef. What few people realize is that *any* type of food can become contaminated. That said, some foods, because of certain characteristics they share, are identified as *potentially hazardous foods.*

What do these foods have in common?

- They are moist.
- They have a somewhat neutral pH.
- They contain protein.
- They have a history of contributing to foodborne illness outbreak in the United States.

According to the Food and Drug Administration's Food Code, a model used by local, state, and federal regulators to develop or update their own food safety regulations, potentially hazardous foods include: (www.fda.gov)

- Milk and milk products
- Meats: beef, lamb, pork
- Poultry
- Eggs
- Raw sprouts
- Shellfish and crustaceans
- Fish
- Cooked potatoes
- Heat-treated, plant-based foods like rice or beans
- Tofu or textured soy protein
- Sliced melons
- Garlic-and-oil mixtures

How Food Becomes Unsafe

Cases of foodborne illness typically involve several factors. Three common factors that contribute to its onset include: time-temperature abuse, poor personal hygiene, and cross contamination.

Keep Hot Foods Hot and Cold Foods Cold! Avoiding Time Temperature Abuse

For microorganisms to grow and multiply, they need the right temperature. If potentially hazardous foods are kept in the temperature danger zone, which is between the temperatures of 41 to 135 degrees Fahrenheit, for four hours or longer, microorganisms can grow to levels high enough to make someone ill. Therefore, foods, especially potentially hazardous foods, should either be kept cold, cooked thoroughly, and then kept hot, if necessary (on a hot buffet, for example).

Dirty Hands = Dirty Food! Avoiding Poor Personal Hygiene

Your mother was right when she told you to wash your hands. Hand washing is one of the most important things that you can do to avoid foodborne illness. Coughing, sneezing, scratching, or picking your face all can contaminate food. To avoid contracting foodborne illness due to poor personal hygiene, insist food handlers wear gloves while preparing your food, hand wash prior to eating, and encourage friends and family to hand wash when eating together. A simple rinse will not do the job. Proper hand washing should last for roughly 20 seconds, or long enough to sing, "Happy Birthday" two times.

Using warm water and soap, create a lather and scrub under nails, in between fingers, and on backs of hands. Next, rinse, and using a paper towel, turn off the water faucet. Finally, dry hands on unused portion of the paper towel.

Microorganisms Can Move From Surface to Surface—Avoiding Cross-Contamination

Cross-contamination results when microorganisms are transferred from one surface to another. This is a major contributing factor behind foodborne illness that you might least expect. Consider the following scenario.

It's a beautiful day and you and your friends want to have a backyard barbeque. You all decide to hit the grocery store and stock up on your favorite grilling foods: ribs, burgers, and hot dogs. You also pick up some sides of coleslaw and potato salad. The food tasted great, the party was fun, and everyone had a good time. Later that night, however, you feel horrible. You've got diarrhea, vomiting and abdominal pain. Immediately, you suspect the burger you ate at the cookout as the culprit. It probably wasn't cooked thoroughly even, although you saw your buddy use a thermometer to measure internal temperature of the burger. Still, you think, it must be the burger. What else could it be?

At this point, it's important to recognize that the burger could very well have been completely cooked. None of that matters, however, if the chef failed to use separate cooking tongs for the raw ground beef patties and the buns. In other words, let's say there was a plate of raw patties waiting for grilling. Using a pair of tongs, your friend grabs them one-by-one and puts them on the hot grill. He cooks them thoroughly; he even measured their internal temperature with a culinary thermometer for safety. Using the same tongs, he grabbed the cooked burgers and put them on a clean plate. Next, he picked ups the buns toasting on the grill (again, using the same tongs) and then placed those on fresh plate.

It's clear that the cook has cross-contaminated the food at least two times. The first time is when he removed the cooked burgers from the grill with the same tongs he used to put them on the grill when they were raw. The second time is when the cook uses the same tongs to remove the toasted buns from the grill. In fact, it wasn't the burger that caused the foodborne illness in this scenario. It was thoroughly cooked. The real culprit is the microorganisms that were cross contaminated during the cooking process.

Steps You Can Take to Avoid Contamination

- Use color-coded cutting boards in your kitchen: red for meats, yellow for poultry, white for fish, and green for produce.
- Avoid rinsing meat/poultry/fish prior to cooking. The cooking process alone will destroy any pathogens present. Rinsing allows the opportunity for contaminated water to splash or cross contaminate on kitchen surfaces.
- After handling raw meat/poultry/fish, wash your hands. Let's say that you have placed raw chicken breasts in a pan to bake. You open the oven and place the pan on a rack to cook. If you did not wash your hands after handling the raw chicken, you have now contaminated the handle of the oven door.
- Have plenty of clean cooking utensils on hand while cooking. Let's say that you are not certain if a piece of meat is completely cooked. And, although you plan to use a thermometer, you want to cut into it to see what color the inside meat is. Once finished, you lay the fork and knife you used on the countertop. Now, not only is the countertop contaminated, but so are the utensils.
- Finally, remember that a food can be cross-contaminated even after it is cooked! Let's say that you remove cooked chicken breasts from the oven. You place them on the counter on a plate to cool for a few minutes. They are a little cooler now, so you begin cutting them into cubes for a chicken salad you are making. While you are cutting though, you scratch an itch on the side of your nose and then finish cutting the remainder of the cooked chicken. Because of the seemingly harmless scratch on the nose, you have now cross-contaminated any microorganisms that might have been present there, such as Staphylococcus.

Recent Foodborne Illness Outbreaks

You don't have to be a food safety expert to have heard about the recent foodborne illness outbreaks in the news. From less well known culprits like spinach, to more commonly known suspects like beef, there has been a rash of outbreaks leaving consumers scared about what to eat and what to avoid.

What Are Foodborne Disease Outbreaks and Why Do They Occur?

The Centers for Disease Control and Prevention (CDC) defines an *outbreak* of foodborne illness as when a group of people consume the same contaminated food and *two or more* of them develop the same illness. It may be a group that ate a meal together somewhere, or it may be a group of people who do not know each other at all, but who all happened to buy and eat the same contaminated item from a grocery store or restaurant.

The CDC identifies that many outbreaks are local in nature. They are recognized when a group of people realize that they all became ill after a common meal, and someone calls the local health department. This type of local outbreak might follow a catered meal at a reception, a pot-luck supper, or eating a meal at an understaffed restaurant on a particularly busy day. However, outbreaks are increasingly being recognized that are more widespread, affect persons in many different places, and are spread out over several weeks.

Some of the Most Common Foodborne Diseases

According to the CDC, the most commonly recognized foodborne illnesses are those caused by the bacteria Campylobacter, Salmonella, and E. coli O157:H7, and by a group of viruses called calicivirus, also known as the Norwalk and Norwalk-like viruses.

Campylobacter is a bacterial pathogen that can cause fever, diarrhea, and abdominal cramps. It is the most commonly identified bacterial cause of diarrheal illness in the world. These bacteria live in the intestines of healthy birds, and most raw poultry meat has Campylobacter on it. Eating undercooked chicken, or other food that has been cross-contaminated with juice drippings from raw chicken, is the most frequent source of this illness.

Salmonella is also a bacterium that is widespread in the intestines of birds, reptiles, and mammals. It can spread to humans via a variety of different foods of animal origin. The illness it causes, salmonellosis, typically includes fever, diarrhea, and abdominal cramps. In persons with poor underlying health or weakened immune systems, it can invade the bloodstream and cause life-threatening infections.

E. coli O157:H7 is a bacterial pathogen that has a reservoir in cattle and other similar animals. Human illness typically follows consumption of food or water that has been contaminated with microscopic amounts of cow feces. The illness it causes is often a severe and bloody diarrhea and painful abdominal cramps, without much fever. In 3 to 5 percent of cases, a complication called hemolytic uremic syndrome (HUS) can occur several weeks after the initial symptoms. This severe complication includes temporary anemia, profuse bleeding, and kidney failure.

Calicivirus, or Norwalk-like virus, is an extremely common cause of foodborne illness, though it is rarely diagnosed, because the laboratory test is not widely available. It causes an acute gastrointestinal illness, usually with more vomiting than diarrhea that resolves within two days. Unlike many foodborne pathogens that have animal reservoirs, it is believed that Norwalk-like viruses spread primarily from one infected person to another. Infected kitchen workers can contaminate a salad or sandwich as they prepare it, if they have the virus on their hands. Infected fishermen have contaminated oysters as they harvested them.

Recent Outbreaks

- In 2003, three people died of Hepatitis A after eating green onions in Pennsylvania. Hundreds more were seriously sickened.
- In 2006, E. coli-contaminated spinach killed three peopled and sickened hundreds.
- In June 2007, there were at least 14 cases of E. coli poisoning because of 5.7 million pounds of tainted beef shipped to 11 different states.
- In May 2008, the USDA recalled 808 lbs of ground beef due to E. coli contamination; and 290 lbs of pork sausage was recalled due to listeria contamination.

For more information or to receive automatic notification of recall updates, visit the USDA's website at: http://www.fsis.usda.gov/Fsis_Recalls/index.asp.

ASSIGNMENT #7

Name: _____

Date: _____

1. Have you or any family member suffered from a foodborne illness?

   - What were the symptoms and effects?
   - What are the most common causes of foodborne illnesses?

_____

_____

_____

_____

_____

_____

_____

_____

_____

_____

_____

_____

_____

_____

_____

_____

2. How would you advise a group of food handlers on avoiding spread of food infections? Explain key messages you would convey to them.

_____

_____

_____

_____

_____

_____

_____

_____

_____

_____

_____

_____

_____

_____

_____

_____

RESOURCES

American Journal of Clinical Nutrition, November 2002 Vol. 76, No. 5, 911–922.

Appleton, Nancy, PhD, Fructose is No Answer For a Sweetener, http://www.mercola.com/2002/jan/5/fructose.htm.

Bryan, F. L. Diseases transmitted by foods. Atlanta: Centers for Disease Control (1982).

Centers for Disease Control and Prevention, U.S. Department of Agriculture, Food and Drug Administration: www.cdc.gov/ncidod/dbmd/diseaseinfo/.

Center for Science in the Public Interest: www.cfsan.fda.gov/~dms/.

Center for Science in the Public Interest; *Outbreak Alert! 2005,* http://www.cspinet.org/foodsafety/.

Centre for Science and Environment: www.cseindia.org.

Environmental Protection Agency Local Drinking Water Reports: www.epa.gov/safewater/dwinfo.htm.

Environmental Protection Agency: Fish advisory 2007: http://www.epa.gov/waterscience/fish/advice/factsheet.html.

Environmental Working Group: *www.ewg.org.*

Fallon, Sally and Mary Enig, *Nourishing Traditions,* New Trends Publishing, Washington DC, 2001, p. 23.

Food and Drug Administration (FDA) Food Code: http://www.cfsan.fda.gov/~dms/fc05-toc.html.

Fortune Magazine: The safety of bottled water http://money.cnn.com/2007/04/24/news/economy/pluggedin_gunther_water.fortune/.

Hartford Advocate News, August 28, 2003.

Hallfrisch, Judith, Metabolic Effects of Dietary Fructose, *FASEB Journal* 4 (June 1990): 2652–2660.

Howard, Brian, *E Magazine,* Sept/Oct 2003, "Message in a Bottle," www.emagazine.com.

Hunter, Beatrice Trum, Confusing Consumers About Sugar Intake, *Consumer's Research* 78, No. 1 (January 1995): 14–17.

Glennon, John, *Water Follies, Groundwater Pumping and the Fate of America's Fresh Waters,* 2002, Island Press.

Natural Resource Defense Council: http://www.nrdc.org/default.asp.

Natural Resources Defense Council: www.nrdc.org/water/drinking/bw/bwinx.asp.

Nestle, M. *What to Eat;* May 2006 by Farrar, Straus and Giroux, LLC.

New York Times Magazine "Power Steer" (March 31, 2002).

NSF Bottled Water program: www.nsf.org.

Organic Trade Association: http://www.ota.com.

PBS/Point of View Borders: www.pbs.org/pov/borders/2004/water.

Schlosser, E. *Fast Food Nation.* Jan 2001 by Mifflin.

Sinclair, U. *The Jungle;* Feb 1906 by Doubleday, Jabber & Company.

United States Department of Agriculture (USDA): http://www.fsis.usda.gov/Fsis_Recalls/index.asp.

OBESITY AND WEIGHT MANAGEMENT

As Americans, we hear a lot about being "overweight" and "obese." In fact, for the first time in several decades, obesity is the second leading cause of preventable death in the United States, and is close to trading places with tobacco use, which is the first leading cause of preventable death in the United States.

Some statistics

- Results from the 2003 to 2004 National Health and Nutrition Examination Survey (NHANES), using measured heights and weights, indicate that an estimated 66 percent of American adults are either overweight or obese.
- Results from the 2003 to 2004 National Health and Nutrition Examination Survey (NHANES), using measured heights and weights, indicate that an estimated 17 percent of children and adolescents ages 2 to 19 years are overweight.
- More than 50 million Americans are currently on a diet, with roughly 5 percent losing weight over the long term.
- Obesity among adults has more than doubled since 1980.
- Less than one-third of Americans meet the federal recommendations to engage in at least 30 minutes of moderate physical activity most days of the week, and 40 percent of adults engage in no physical activity at all.

UNITED STATES OBESITY TRENDS, 1985 TO 2007

During the past 20 years, there has been a dramatic increase in obesity in the United States.

According to the Centers for Disease Control and Prevention, in 2007, only one state (Colorado) had a prevalence of obesity less than 20 percent. Thirty states had a prevalence equal to or greater than 25 percent; three of these states (Alabama, Mississippi and Tennessee) had a prevalence of obesity equal to or greater than 30 percent.

2007 State Obesity Rates

State	%	State	%	State	%	State	%
Alabama	30.3	Illinois	24.9	Montana	21.8	Rhode Island	21.4
Alaska	27.5	Indiana	26.8	Nebraska	26.0	South Carolina	28.4
Arizona	25.4	Iowa	26.9	Nevada	24.1	South Dakota	26.2
Arkansas	28.7	Kansas	26.9	New Hampshire	24.4	Tennessee	30.1
California	22.6	Kentucky	27.4	New Jersey	23.5	Texas	28.1
Colorado	18.7	Louisiana	29.8	New Mexico	24.0	Utah	21.8
Connecticut	21.2	Maine	24.8	New York	25.0	Vermont	21.3
Delaware	27.4	Maryland	25.4	North Carolina	28.0	Virginia	24.3
Washington DC	21.8	Massachusetts	21.3	North Dakota	26.5	Washington	25.3
Florida	23.6	Michigan	27.7	Ohio	27.5	West Virginia	29.5
Georgia	28.2	Minnesota	25.6	Oklahoma	28.1	Wisconsin	24.7
Hawaii	21.4	Mississippi	32.0	Oregon	25.5	Wyoming	23.7
Idaho	24.5	Missouri	27.5	Pennsylvania	27.1		

Source: U.S. Obesity Trends 1985–2007 www.cdc.gov

MEASURING OVERWEIGHT AND OBESITY

There are a few different ways to assess whether or not a person is overweight or obese. Many people rely on a traditional scale at home or at the doctor's office, but in some cases, these numbers can be misleading.

Height and Weight Charts

Height and weight tables were originally developed and heavily used by life insurance actuaries. An actuary determines a person's eligibility for insurance based on different health factors, weight being one of them. You can imagine the slight conflict of interest. In other words, when a huge insurance company creates a height-weight table, it is in its best financial interest to establish the weight ranges on the low end. Why is this? It means because you do not meet the strict weight requirements, you must pay more money to be insured.

Waist Circumference

Waist circumference is defined as the perimeter around your natural waist, where your belly button falls, not your hips. Assessing this number provides clues about a person's health that charts and tables cannot. Most importantly, it indicates where you are carrying any excess weight. People tend to fall into one of two categories:

1. Pear   *or*   2. Apple

In general, men tend to be apples, whereas women tend to be pears. Once a woman hits menopause, however, she may start to accumulate body fat through the abdominal region and have more of an apple appearance instead of a pear. This is due in large part to the decrease in estrogen, which dictates where fat is stored.

What Does It Mean to Be an *Apple* or a *Pear*?

Pears tend to accumulate any excess body fat in the hip, buttock, and thigh region whereas apples tend to accumulate it through the abdominal area. As it relates to health, it is always preferable to store excess body fat in the hip, buttock, and thigh region rather than the abdominal area. Why is this?

By the time your tailor's tape says your waistline is larger than 39 inches, you may already be on the road to diabetes or heart disease. This holds true for both men and women (Wahrenberg, 2005). Excessive abdominal fat is serious because it places you at greater risk for developing obesity-related conditions, such as type 2 diabetes, high blood cholesterol, high triglycerides, high blood pressure, and coronary artery disease.

More specifically, it is recommended that men maintain a stricter waist circumference of 35″ or less and women maintain a waist circumference of 32.5″ or less (Roizen & Oz, 2006).

Why? Wahrenberg's research found that half of all men and women with waistlines of one meter or more—that's 39.37 inches or more in the United States—already have insulin resistance, where the body's cells are less responsive to the hormone insulin. On the other hand, very few people with smaller waists have developed this dangerous condition.

How to Measure Your Waist Size and Waist-to-Hip Ratio

To measure your waist size (circumference), place a tape measure around your bare abdomen above your hip bones around your belly button. Be sure that the tape is snug, but does not compress your skin, and is parallel to the floor. Relax, exhale, and measure your waist.

Remember, where you carry body fat is just as important as how much you carry. People who tend to accumulate fat around the waist (apple shape) have a higher risk of heart disease, diabetes, and high blood pressure than those who carry excess weight on the hips and thighs (pear shape).

In addition to measuring your waist circumference, you can calculate your waist-to-hip ratio (WHR). This is another way to determine if the weight in your abdomen exceeds that of your thighs.

WHR is the measurement of your waist divided by the measurement of your hips. Measure your waist at the level of your belly button as instructed above. A WHR greater than 1 for men and 0.8 for women is considered unfavorable.

Body Mass Index (BMI)

Today, most physicians and other health professionals rely on a type of measurement called body mass index (BMI). Body mass index is a method of measuring a person's *degree* of overweight or obesity. It is thought to be a more sensitive indicator than traditional height-weight charts (Drummond & Brefere, 2004).

To determine your BMI, you must know your weight in pounds and your height in inches. For example, a person who is 5′6″ (66″) and weighs 136lbs. has a BMI of 22.

BMI	19	20	21	22	23	24	25	26	27	28	29	30	31	32	33	34	35
Height (inches)								Body Weight (pounds)									
58	91	96	100	105	110	115	119	124	129	134	138	143	148	153	158	162	167
59	94	99	104	109	114	119	124	128	133	138	143	148	153	158	163	168	173
60	97	102	107	112	118	123	128	133	138	143	148	153	158	163	168	174	179
61	100	106	111	116	122	127	132	137	143	148	153	158	164	169	174	180	185
62	104	109	115	120	126	131	136	142	147	153	158	164	169	175	180	186	191
63	107	113	118	124	130	135	141	146	152	158	163	169	175	180	186	191	197
64	110	116	122	128	134	140	145	151	157	163	169	174	180	186	192	197	204
65	114	120	126	132	138	144	150	156	162	168	174	180	186	192	198	204	210
66	118	124	130	136	142	148	155	161	167	173	179	186	192	198	204	210	216
67	121	127	134	140	146	153	159	166	172	178	185	191	198	204	211	217	223
68	125	131	138	144	151	158	164	171	177	184	190	197	203	210	216	223	230
69	128	135	142	149	155	162	169	176	182	189	196	203	209	216	223	230	236
70	132	139	146	153	160	167	174	181	188	195	202	209	216	222	229	236	243
71	136	143	150	157	165	172	179	186	193	200	208	215	222	229	236	243	250
72	140	147	154	162	169	177	184	191	199	206	213	221	228	235	242	250	258
73	144	151	159	166	174	182	189	197	204	212	219	227	235	242	250	257	265
74	148	155	163	171	179	186	194	202	210	218	225	233	241	249	256	264	272
75	152	160	168	176	184	192	200	208	216	224	232	240	248	256	264	272	279
76	156	164	172	180	189	197	205	213	221	230	238	246	254	263	271	279	287

Source: National Heart, Lung, and Blood Institute (NHBLI) of the U.S. Department of Health and Human Services

Understanding Your BMI

There are four main BMI Categories:

1. **Underweight** = <18.5
2. **Normal weight** = 18.5 to 24.9
3. **Overweight** = 25 to 29.9
4. **Obesity** = BMI of 30 or greater

Overweight Versus Obese

What is the difference between being overweight and being obese? Overweight and obesity are both labels for ranges of weight that are greater than what is generally considered healthy for a given height. The terms also identify ranges of weight that have been shown to increase the likelihood of certain diseases and other health problems (Centers for Disease Control and Prevention, 2007).

For adults, overweight and obesity ranges are determined by using weight and height to calculate body mass index. An adult who has a BMI between 25 and 29.9 is considered overweight whereas an adult who has a BMI of 30 or higher is considered obese.

If you have been thinking about your current weight, it may be because you've noticed a change in how your clothes fit. Or maybe you have been told by a health care professional that you have high blood pressure or high cholesterol and that your weight could be a contributing factor. The first step is to determine whether or not your current weight is healthy. BMI is just one way to determine whether your weight is a healthy one.

Body Fat Percentage

One of the best ways to really determine your "fatness" is to have your body composition assessed. The human body is made up of water (roughly 60 percent), bone mineral, organs and other tissue/viscera, muscle, and fat. When a person steps on a scale, the number he or she sees is greatly influenced by factors such as water retention, hormone fluctuation and the weight of the fecal matter in the intestines. If you are going to weigh yourself, do so no more than one time per week (unless your doctor instructs otherwise), after a bowel movement, and before eating or drinking anything.

Have you ever noticed how two people whose heights and weights are the same can look so different? For example, let's say that in front of you stand two women who have the exact same statistics:

* Both are 5'8"
* Both are 35 years old
* Both weigh 145 lbs
* Both have a medium bone frame

When you look at both of these women, even though they share all of the above statistics, they look very different. One of the women looks much smaller than the other. What's going on?

The answer is that they have different body composition. At this point, it is important to recognize that muscle and adipose (fat) are two different types of tissue. Adipose tissue is like marshmallow, oozy and fluffy. It takes up a lot of space. Muscle tissue, on the other hand, is dense and tight. It takes up very little space. Muscle, however, does not weigh more than adipose. What differs though is their density. Because muscle tissue is so dense, it takes up less space than adipose tissue making a person's appearance smaller or leaner.

The "Skinny Fat Person"

Some obesity researchers now believe that the internal fat surrounding vital organs like the heart, liver, or pancreas, invisible to the naked eye, could be as dangerous as the more obvious external fat that bulges underneath the skin. In other words, being "thin" does not necessarily mean you are lean. A skinny-fat person, sometimes referred to as "thin outside, fat inside" (TOFI), typically has very little lean muscle mass and a lot of adipose tissue, which makes their total body weight appear normal.

In fact, fat, active people, sometimes called "fit and fat," can be healthier than their skinny, sedentary counterparts. Normal weight people who are sedentary and unfit are at much higher risk for developing disease than obese persons who are active and fit. How can this be?

Obesity researchers believe that people who are not overweight but still have a high percentage of body fat may have more inflammation in their bodies. These people are often referred to as "normal-weight obese" because of their high body fat percentage.

When researchers took blood samples from research subjects, they found those who were overweight or obese had the highest levels of inflammatory chemicals, LDL ("bad") cholesterol, and triglycerides (a type of blood fat). However, the "normal-weight obese" women also had higher levels of inflammatory chemicals than those with both a normal BMI and lower body fat. These findings indicate that the normal-weight women with high body fat "were in an early inflammatory state," because body fat is thought to release inflammatory chemicals, according to the researchers (De Lorenzo et al., 2007). Chronically high levels of inflammation have been associated with a host of health problems, including heart disease and arthritis.

Research also shows that people who maintain their weight through diet rather than exercise are likely to have major deposits of internal fat, even if they are otherwise slim. Typically, thin people may falsely assume that because they are not overweight, they are healthy.

In reality, a skinny fat person may have a "normal" weight, but this does not make them immune to diabetes or other risk factors for heart disease.

Skinny fat people, who are fat on the inside, are essentially on the threshold of being obese. They eat too many fatty, sugary foods, and exercise too little to work it off, but they are not eating enough to actually be overweight.

Most experts believe that being of normal weight is an indicator of good health, and that BMI is a reliable measurement. BMI won't give you the exact indication of where fat is, but it can be a useful clinical tool. Still, getting a body composition assessment would be a better indicator of body fat percentage.

MEASURING BODY FAT PERCENTAGE

Two popular and often used techniques for measuring body fat include:

Skinfold Calipers

Skinfold calipers are a type of "old school" measurement that looks like kitchen tongs. They are used by "pinching" a fold of fat on different regions of the body such as the bicep, tricep, subscapular, above the hip bone, and sometimes on the calf. There is room for error, however, if the person performing the assessment "pinches" the skin fold too hard. This makes the person appear "leaner" than they really are. It's important that the technician (usually a personal trainer, dietician, or other health professional) measure the sites three separate times and then average his or her findings to account for human error.

Bio-electrical Impedance Analysis (BIA)

Bioelectrical impedance is measured when a very small electrical signal carried by water and fluids is passed through the body. Impedance is greatest in fat tissue (this interferes with the passing of the electrical current), which contains only 10 to 20 percent water, whereas fat-free mass, which contains 70 to 75 percent water, allows the signal to pass much more easily.

If a person is dehydrated, the amount of fat tissue can be overestimated. Factors that can affect hydration include not drinking enough fluids, drinking too much caffeine or alcohol, exercising or eating just before measuring, taking certain prescription drugs or diuretics, illness, or a woman's menstrual cycle. Measuring under consistent conditions is important to get accurate results with this method.

Tips to Improve Body Composition

- Commit to cardiovascular exercise at a vigorous intensity at least 3 days per week, preferably four or five. Interval training is great for reducing body fat and maintaining lean muscle tissue. Interval training is short bursts of intense cardiovascular exercise followed by rest and recovery periods of lower intensity work. For example, if you are on a treadmill, after warming up, you might sprint for 30 to 45 seconds and then recover by jogging or walking for 2 to 3 minutes. This cycle would then be repeated 4 to 5 times in a 30-minute session.

- Include weight training 2 to 3 times per week. Start with large muscle exercises that work areas such as the back, legs, arms, and chest. Start slowly, but work up to lifting a weight that is challenging. If you can easily lift a given weight 15 repetitions or more, consider increasing the weight. Remember, building muscle means making the body appear smaller and toned. Try weight training followed by a shorter cardio session. This offers the benefit of maximum strength for lifting and continued fat burning during the cardio.

- Eat protein with every meal, and try to eat every three hours. Protein is the building block of muscle, and it is essential for tissue repair.

- Round out your meals with complex carbohydrates like whole grains, fruits, vegetables, and legumes, and always eat within 45 minutes after exercise.

- Manage stress to reduce levels of the stress hormone cortisol, which can increase abdominal fat and muscle breakdown. Practice meditation, stretching, and/or yoga to help decrease stress levels.

CAUSES OF OBESITY

Many think of fat as greasy blobs stored under the skin, but it is now widely accepted that it behaves more like an active organ, constantly changing and sending out hormones that affect your mood, ability to think clearly, and fertility levels.

The fat just underneath the skin is called subcutaneous fat. Internal fat (the kind sitting around the abdomen and surrounding vital organs) is referred to as visceral fat.

Fat cells are kind of like "chemical factories" producing other substances and causing inflammation, which can cause long-term harm. They contribute to diabetes, heart disease, high blood pressure, strokes, and other illnesses, including some cancers.

If you eat more food calories than you burn, the excess is stored in your fat cells. How much fat a person has reflects both the number and the size of the fat cells (Whitney & Rolfes, 2002). During periods of rapid growth, such as puberty, fat cells increase significantly (Bray, 1992).

The only way to get rid of fat cells is through a cosmetic procedure, such as liposuction. In other words, fat cells can expand in size. And once they reach their maximum size, they may also divide. When you lose weight, the number of fat cells remains the same. They simply shrink in size, but do not go away.

As you put on more weight, the cells grow bigger, sending out messages to nearby cells, which start to divide to produce more fat cells. A lean adult has 40 billion fat cells; an obese adult has two to three times that.

Body shape is often governed by genetic factors. When both parents are overweight, their children have a high likelihood of also being overweight. People shaped like apples, carrying excess weight in the abdomen, are more at risk than those built like pears, who deposit fat in the hips, thighs, and backsides. Women tend to fall into the latter category. Constant dieting may interfere with the way the body lays down fat, and there is evidence that this will increase visceral fat.

Overeating is a major factor behind obesity. Food portion sizes have increased since the 1970s. Today, foods are king-sized, big-slam, and super-sized. With more Americans eating out and grabbing food on-the-go, it is no surprise that they are taking in more food calories than they need without realizing it.

For many people, eating is an action that occurs in response to psychological factors like boredom, anxiety, stress, anger, sadness, and happiness. When a person regularly eats for reasons other than biological hunger, that is, they are eating to satisfy their psychological appetite, they are likely to have a weight problem. Think about it. An animal in the wild will hunt its food and eat in response to the biological of hunger. It does not do this, however, because it had a bad day at work. Nor will it overeat. Once it is satisfied, the animal will cease eating.

Modern technology has replaced muscle activity at home and at work, which means we move less today than a century ago. Technology has contributed to a sedentary lifestyle among the American population. Picture the typical American's work day: They rise after sleeping (sedentary), sit down and eat breakfast (sedentary), and then get into their car to drive to work (sedentary). Once at work, they sit behind their desk in front of a computer (sedentary). Once work day is finished, the person drives home (sedentary), eats dinner (sedentary), and relaxes in front of the television (sedentary) before going to bed (sedentary).

If you ask the average American whether or not they are sedentary, most will cry foul. However, they are confusing being *busy* with being *active*. Many Americans lead very hectic lives working, taking care of children and other family members, and going to school. All of these activities give the *perception* of a lifestyle that is anything but sedentary. Unless a person is elevating their heart rate through physical activity multiple times a week for a period of time, they are, in fact, sedentary.

Two hormones are now thought to be factors behind overweight and obesity. One is leptin, which helps suppress appetite and promote energy expenditure. Leptin is made in the fat cells. Logically, you would question that obese people have a lot of leptin and, therefore, should be lean. It is true that obese people do have a lot of leptin; however, it is thought that leptin's actions are ineffective in obese people. They appear to have a resistance to it.

Ghrelin, on the other hand, is a hormone produced mainly by cells lining the stomach and cells of the pancreas that stimulates appetite (Inui, 2004). Ghrelin levels increase before meals and decrease after meals. It is considered the counterpart of the hormone leptin. Ghrelin does not cause obesity, but scientists think controlling it might help us get our weight back in balance. Not surprisingly, in some bariatric procedures, the level of ghrelin is reduced in patients, thus causing satiation before it would normally occur.

Disease States Associated with Overweight and Obesity

The bulk of diseases in the United States would be eradicated if obesity rates would normalize. The following are associated with being overweight or obese:

- Hypertension (high blood pressure)
- Osteoarthritis (a degeneration of cartilage and its underlying bone within a joint)
- Dyslipidemia (for example, high total cholesterol or high levels of triglycerides)
- Type 2 diabetes
- Coronary heart disease
- Stroke
- Gallbladder disease
- Sleep apnea and respiratory problems
- Some cancers (endometrial, breast, and colon)

Two of the Healthy People 2010's national health objectives are (1) to reduce the prevalence of overweight and obesity among adults to less than 15 percent and (2) to reduce the prevalence of obesity among children and adolescents to less than 5 percent.

CALCULATING ENERGY NEEDS

Three main components determine your body's energy expenditure. Adding these three components together, basal metabolic rate, energy expended during physical activity, and the thermic effect of food is the most accurate way of determining how many calories your body requires each day.

1. *Basal Metabolic Rate (BMR):* Most of the body's energy, about 60 to 70 percent, goes to supporting the ongoing metabolic work of the body's cells. This includes such activities as heart beat, respiration, and maintaining body temperature.
2. *Physical Activity:* Physical activity has a significant impact on energy expenditure and contributes roughly 20 to 30 percent to the body's total energy output. In other words, the more physically active you are, the more food calories you require to maintain your current weight.
3. *Thermic Effect of Food:* This is the energy expended by the body simply to digest and absorb food. You burn roughly 5 to 10 percent due to the thermic effect of food.

Below is a simple formula to determine your daily calorie needs that takes into account all three of the above components.

For sedentary people: Weight × 14 = estimated calories/day

For moderately active people: Weight × 17 = estimated calories/day

For active people: Weight × 20 = estimated calories/day

"Moderately active" is defined as 3 to 4 aerobic sessions per week. "Active" is defined as 5 to 7 aerobic sessions per week.

To lose weight, you must create a caloric deficit preferably through both diet and exercise. It is recommended that you aim to lose one to two pounds per week. One pound of body fat contains 3,500 calories. So, if you wanted to lose one pound of body fat in one week, you would need to subtract 250 food calories from the above number you got and burn 250 calories most days of the week through physical activity. This would roughly create a 500 calorie per day deficit. 500×7 days in a week = 3,500.

Example:

> Jane is 5'6" and weighs 172 pounds. She is busy but not active and, therefore, realizes that she is sedentary.
>
> $172 \times 14 = 2,408$
>
> Jane is consuming roughly 2,400 calories to maintain her current weight of 172 pounds. In order to lose weight, she will need to cut her food intake by 250 calories per day and burn extra calories through exercise. A 45-minute power walk would burn roughly 250 calories.
>
> So, instead of eating her normal 2,400 calories, Jane will eat roughly 2,150 (2,400 – 250 = 2,150). Instead of being sedentary, Jane will work out 4 to 5 days per week or more increasing her energy expenditure. This will result in a one pound weight loss per week.

PHYSICAL ACTIVITY

As previously mentioned, people who combine diet with exercise tend to not only have lower rates of visceral fat, but also are more likely to maintain weight loss and have improved mood due to the psychological benefits of exercise. So, how much is enough?

It is generally acknowledged that you should work out at least three to five times per week. An exercise program should include both cardiovascular activities (e.g., running, stair-climbing, fast walking) and strength training.

Cardio should be done for 20 to 60 minutes. A person who has been sedentary should start slowly. Over time, stamina and cardiorespiratory function will increase, and the person will be able to go longer.

Strength training should be done 2 to 3 times per week with a focus on the major muscle groups: back, chest, thighs, gluteals, arms, and shoulders. A weight should be challenging enough that you cannot do any more than 15 repetitions. If you can do more than that using proper form, you should increase the weight that you are using.

RESOURCES

Bray, G. A. (1992). Pathophysiology of obesity. *American Journal of Clinical Nutrition,* Vol 55: 488S–494S.

Centers For Disease Control and Prevention. U.S. Obesity Trends 1985–2007: www.cdc.org.

De Lorenzo, A. et al. (2007). Normal-weight obese syndrome: early inflammation? *American Journal of Clinical Nutrition,* Vol. 85, No. 1: 40–45.

Drummond, K. E., & Brefere, L. M. (2004). *Nutrition for foodservice and culinary professionals,* 5th Edition. John Wiley & Sons, Inc.

Inui A. et al. (2004). Ghrelin, appetite, and gastric motility: the emerging role of the stomach as an endocrine organ. *Federation of American Societies for Experimental Biology Journal.* 18 (3): 439–56.

National Health and Nutrition Examination Survey (NHANES), 2003 to 2004. National Center for Health Statistics: http://www.cdc.gov/nchs/about/major/nhanes/nhanes2003–2004/nhanes03_04.htm.

Roizen, M. F., & Oz, M. C. (2006). *You on a diet: The owner's manual for waist management.* Simon & Schuster, Inc.

U.S. Department of Health and Human Services. Healthy People 2010. 2nd ed. With Understanding and Improving Health and Objectives for Improving Health. 2 vols. Washington, DC: U.S. Government Printing Office, November 2000.

Wahrenberg, H. (2005) *British Medical Journal,* Online First edition, April 15.

Whitney, E. N., & Rolfes, S. R. (2002). *Understanding Nutrition,* 9th Edition. Wadsworth Thomson Learning.

MYTHS AND MISCONCEPTIONS

9

Fads abound in the field of nutrition and, naturally, so do a plethora of myths and misconceptions about what to eat, what not to eat, how to eat, and so on. The growing relevance of nutrition and its relationship to disease prevention has piqued the interested of many "arm chair" nutritionists. That is, many lay people have become well versed on basic nutrition principles. The problem, however, is that while although may have some things right, they often have many things wrong.

Many misperceptions exist within the field of nutrition and probably will only get worse as time goes on. The following myths and misperceptions have been compiled by the authors over many years of clinical practice and academic experience. Students continue to be a source of inspiration behind these myths often debunking them on their own once they have taken class! To become a critical consumer, you must read food labels and nutritional claims carefully. Eventually, you will be able to food shop and eat with confidence!

MYTHS AND MISCONCEPTIONS

Eating Sugar Causes Diabetes

Hands down, when teaching about diabetes, the eating-sugar-causes-diabetes myth is a repeat offender. It seems that people have interpreted the notion that too much sugar in the blood is what causes diabetes, when in, fact, elevated blood sugar is really the *symptom* of a greater underlying problem. Let's review what is going on when a person has diabetes. First, some definitions are required:

Hormone:

A chemical "messenger"; delivers a product from point A to point B.

Insulin:

Hormone responsible for delivering glucose from point A: the bloodstream, to Point B: the body's cells.

Pancreas:

Endocrine organ responsible for secreting the hormone insulin.

There are two main types of diabetes: type 1 and type 2.

Type 1 is an autoimmune disease, one in which your lifestyle behaviors did not contribute to the onset of the illness. Typically people diagnosed with type 1 diabetes are under 25 years old. This type used to be referred to as "juvenile onset." With this type of diabetes, certain cells of the pancreas, called beta cells, which are responsible for making insulin, do not function. Insulin must be injected daily for life.

Type 2 diabetes is the result of lifestyle behaviors, such as being overweight or obese, as well as being sedentary. Old age can also be a cause of type 2 diabetes. In very rare cases, trauma or injury to the body can also contribute to the onset of type 2 diabetes. With type 2 diabetes, the pancreas does work and is manufacturing insulin. However, the body's cells are "resistant" to it because of being overweight/obesity/sedentary lifestyle, etc.

When you eat foods that contain carbohydrates (grains, fruits, veggies, legumes), you experience a normal rise in blood sugar levels (glucose). Insulin comes along (once the pancreas is alerted to the rise in blood sugar) and carries some of the sugar from the meal or snack in the bloodstream to the body's cells, where it can be used as energy. A person with type 1 diabetes must inject the necessary insulin. In a person with type 2 diabetes, the insulin is secreted and carries the sugar (from the bloodstream) to the body's cells, but the cells will not accept the sugar. They are *resistant* to the insulin. In other words, the cells don't respond to the insulin. As a result, the sugar has no where to go (i.e., it cannot enter the cells like it is supposed to) and blood sugar stays elevated. This elevation in blood sugar sends *another* signal to the pancreas to produce even more insulin, so the whole process can be attempted once more. Again, the same result happens: the cells are insulin resistant. Eventually, the pancreas grows tired of sending out insulin and sputters out. Only through proper diet and vigorous exercise will the cells become responsive to insulin again.

So, if you have diabetes, you must watch your sugar and carbohydrate intake to properly manage your blood sugar levels. However, if you do not have diabetes, sugar intake will not cause you to develop the disease. The main risk factors for type 2 diabetes are a diet high in calories, being overweight, and a sedentary lifestyle.

Eating Fat Is Bad, Especially If You Want to Lose Weight

One myth that just will not go away is that if you eat fat, you will be fat. It is a long-held nutrition myth that all fats are bad. But the fact is, we all need fat. Let's recap what fat does:

- Cushions organs
- Acts as an insulator (helps regulate body temperature)
- Helps transport fat-soluble vitamins: A, D, E, K
- Aid nerve transmission
- Help maintain cell membrane integrity
- Help promote satiety (i.e., keeps you feeling satisfied longer in between meals so you're less likely to snack mindlessly)

Not all fats are created equal. Some fats can actually help promote good health, whereas others can clog blood vessels and cause inflammation. It is important to remember that all fats contain 9 calories per gram consumed. They are very energy dense. Remember, saturated fats are typically solid at room temperature and come from the animal kingdom with the exception of tropical oils. Unsaturated fats are typically liquid at room temperature and come from the plant kingdom, with the exception of seafood, like fish. Let's recap our fats:

Unsaturated fats are healthy:
- Olive oil
- Canola oil
- Fatty fish like sardines, halibut, salmon, bluefish, mackerel
- Flaxseed
- Nuts like walnuts
- Soy found in tofu
- Avocado

Saturated fats are unhealthy:
- Lard
- Butter
- Tropical oils like coconut oil, cocoa butter, palm oil
- Marbling on cuts of beef, pork, lamb
- Skin on poultry
- Processed foods like cookies, cakes, candies and chips

Trans fats:
- Processed foods like cookies, cakes, crackers, candy, cereals, and breads.
- Look for the words *partially hydrogenated.* If you see these words, it indicates that trans fats are present in the food product.

Remember, if you eat more food calories than your body needs, you store them as body fat. It does not matter where those calories come from (fat or carbohydrate or protein). If you eat more than you need, you store it as fat.

Carbohydrates Are "Fattening"

This is inherently false because carbohydrate-rich foods contain little, if any, lipid. It is not until we *add* a lipid that they become fattening, for example, cream cheese or butter to your bagel, alfredo sauce or pesto to your pasta, sour cream, and cheese to your potato.

When people go on a low-carbohydrate diet, they often do lose weight. But not for the reasons you think. Many low-carbohydrate diets actually do not provide sufficient carbohydrates to your body for daily maintenance; therefore, your body will begin to burn stored carbohydrates (glycogen) for energy. When your body starts burning glycogen, water is released. In fact, for every gram of carbohydrate, a molecule of water is attached to it. That drastic initial drop of weight at the beginning of a low-carbohydrate diet is mostly the water that you lose as a result of burning glycogen. So, you have lost water weight, *not* body fat.

The fact is, to lose body fat, you must take in fewer calories than your body needs plus exercise. A low-carbohydrate diet gives the perception that you are eating a lot. This is because you are usually eating "forbidden" foods like butter, mayonnaise, fatty meats, creamy salad dressings, and cheese. In reality, low-carbohydrate diets tend to be lower in calorie than traditional diets, thus the weight loss. Here is an example. Let's say today you are *not* on a low carbohydrate diet. You and a friend decide to eat out at a steakhouse. Your dinner begins with bread from the breadbasket. Next, you have an appetizer followed by the entrée of a steak, loaded baked potato, and a vegetable side. For dessert, you eat a slice of carrot cake. All of this is washed down by a glass of red wine.

Now, let's say that tomorrow I *am* on a low-carbohydrate diet. Look at the above meal. What exactly will I be eating? Bread? No. Appetizer? Maybe. Steak? Yes. Potato? No. Veggie side? Maybe. Carrot cake? No. Red wine? No.

The problem with avoiding carbohydrates long term is that it becomes very difficult to maintain. So while you initially lose weight, many people regain the weight and more once they start eating carbohydrates again.

Brown Sugar Is Healthier Than White Sugar

People consistently believe this myth. The fact is, however, sugar is sugar is sugar is sugar. It does not matter whether you eat white sugar or brown sugar or raw sugar. To your body it is all the same thing. And, chemically, it is. It is all made of:

Fructose + Glucose

In fact, the brown sugar sold at grocery stores is actually white granulated sugar with added molasses.

The main reason that there are so many different types of sugar is strictly for baking purposes. Brown sugar, for example, has a high moisture content and, therefore, will make quick breads and cakes more moist. At the end of the day, however, there is no health benefit to selecting one sugar over another. A baking benefit, yes. A health benefit, no.

The one exception to the "sugar is sugar is sugar is sugar" rule is something called high fructose corn syrup. The following is an excerpt from the *San Francisco Chronicle*. Nationally recognized nutrition expert Marion Nestle answers readers' questions in a column titled, Food Matters. This question and answer is specifically about high fructose corn syrup (September 24, 2008).

Q: What is the difference, metabolically speaking, between high-fructose corn syrup and other carbohydrate-based sweeteners (sucrose, fructose, honey, and so on)?

A: From what I hear these days, high-fructose corn syrup (HFCS) is widely perceived as the new trans fat, something to be avoided at all costs. But, stop: HFCS is not poison. It is just sugar in liquid form, differing from common table sugar (sucrose) mainly in how it affects the texture of foods.

I can see why HFCS seems like a nutritional villain: It is a marker for junk foods. Cheaper than sucrose, it turns up in all kinds of processed foods, particularly soft drinks. And there is nearly as much of it in the food supply as sucrose—56 pounds per year per person versus 62 pounds for table sugar.

In its new advertising campaign, the Corn Refiners Association says of HFCS, "Truth is, it's nutritionally the same as table sugar." Truth is, I'd call it almost the same.

Sucrose is a double sugar made of two single sugars—glucose (50 percent) and fructose (50 percent)—stuck together. HFCS also contains glucose and fructose, but the sugars are already separated and their percentages differ slightly. Because sucrose is quickly split by digestive enzymes, the body can hardly tell them apart. For the record, glucose is blood sugar, fructose is fruit sugar, and honey contains both.

The processing of sucrose involves boiling it down from sugar cane or beets, and washing, clarifying, filtering and drying the syrup. HFCS starts out as corn, of course, and you, too, can do what the makers of the indie movie, "King Corn" (2007), demonstrated in my favorite scene.

First, extract the starch. Use enzymes to break down the starch to glucose and to convert some of the glucose to fructose. Then do a bunch of refining, separation and evaporation steps. The resulting syrup is 55 percent fructose, with the rest composed of glucose or undigested starch pieces. The HFCS used in soft drinks has a bit more fructose than sucrose—55 percent as opposed to 50 percent.

Whether this 5 percent difference matters at all depends on whether you are a metabolic optimist or pessimist.

If you are an optimist, you are happy that fructose—unlike glucose—does not stimulate the release of insulin, and in small amounts can be a useful sweetener for people with diabetes.

If you are a pessimist, you will fret that fructose is preferentially metabolized to fat, raising the possibility that HFCS—or any other source of fructose (but we won't worry about fruit)—could have something to do with current obesity trends.

HFCS entered our food supply in the mid 1960s, but did not really come into its own until farm subsidies encouraged farmers to grow as much corn as possible. In 1981, at the dawn of the obesity era, the United States food supply provided 23 pounds of HFCS per person per year, along with 79 pounds of sucrose—102 pounds total.

Today, the balance is 56 to 62 (118 pounds), with the increase entirely due to HFCS. Guilt by association! Glucose corn syrups and honey add up to yet another 18 pounds, but their use has not changed much over time. All told, the food supply provides a third of a pound a day of HFCS and sucrose combined, which works out to about 600 calories a day per person, just from these two sources.

Note that these are available calories, not necessarily those eaten. Availability refers to sugars produced, plus imports, less exports. Even so, people who drink sodas all day long can get a substantial portion of their daily calories from HFCS. Like other sugars, HFCS supplies calories but is devoid of nutrients.

Although only about 6 percent of U.S. corn is used to make corn sweeteners, it is 6 percent of a large number. Corn production is subsidized, and subsidies encourage greater production. Until recently, subsidies drove the cost of corn sweeteners well below that of sucrose, which gets price supports. With corn now going for ethanol, HFCS is more expensive and has less of a price advantage.

Indeed, some food companies have already replaced HFCS with sucrose and are advertising their products as "HFCS-free." At least one grocery chain has said it will no longer carry products containing HFCS. Such events, along with concerns about the metabolic effects of fructose, saddle the Corn Refiners with a challenge—how to convince the American public that HFCS is no worse than any other sugar.

Their methods? First, they successfully petitioned the Food and Drug Administration to allow HFCS to be labeled "natural." Despite the many steps required to process cornstarch into HFCS, the FDA granted their request. Why? Because in processing the enzymes are fixed to a column and the sugars do not come in contact with the synthetic fixing agents. I'm not kidding about this.

Next, the Corn Refiners funded a $30 million counterattack. If you missed the full-page newspaper ads, take a look at the web site, www.sweetsurprise.com.

HFCS has a big public relations problem, but I don't get this campaign. Since when is insulting the intelligence of critics an effective marketing strategy?

I cannot decide which aspects of the campaign are most offensive: The videos of inarticulate critics insulted by their HFCS-savvy friends? The slogans ("HFCS has no artificial ingredients")? The quiz questions ("Which of the following sweeteners is considered a natural food ingredient: HFCS, honey, sugar, or all of the above")? Or the irrelevant take-home message ("As registered dietitians recommend, keep enjoying the foods you love, just do it in moderation")?

I'm not a registered dietitian and maybe that is why I think moderation doesn't work for HFCS. Yes, HFCS has a place in the American diet and sometimes has cooking advantages over sucrose. And the research is still out on whether HFCS differs from sucrose metabolically. But the most sensible approach to HFCS and to sugars in general is not moderation. It is, "Eat less."

Eating Eggs or Shrimp Raise Blood Cholesterol

There is a growing body of evidence demonstrating that the majority of people will have relatively small cholesterol changes in response to changes in dietary cholesterol intake. In other words, eating dietary cholesterol (particularly rich in eggs and shrimp) has less of an effect on cholesterol levels than consuming foods high in saturated and trans fats. What becomes essential for effective interventions to lower cholesterol levels is an overall lowering of saturated and trans fat intake and increase in vigorous physical activity most days of the week. The majority of data available shows that the addition of eggs (at 2 per day) to the diet of healthy people has little effect on plasma cholesterol levels (Ginsberg et al., 1995; Ferrier et al. 1995; Knopp et al. 1997).

The same is true for shrimp and other seafood. Dietary cholesterol found in shrimp and other seafood has little effect on blood cholesterol in most people. Saturated fats and trans fatty acids are the most important factors that raise blood cholesterol.

Keep in mind that when people consume shrimp or other seafood, it is often fried in an unhealthy fat or "dipped" in butter. Implementing a healthy cooking technique is vital to ensuring a lower intake of saturated fat, which is a contributor to elevated blood cholesterol.

Nuts Are Too Fattening!

It is true that nuts are very high in fat and, therefore, quite high in calories. One ounce of walnuts, for example, which is about a small handful, contains 183 calories (USDA's National Nutrient Database for Standard Reference). The key with eating nuts is to do so in moderation. They are very easy to overeat and, as a result, take in a lot of extra calories. Still, nuts can be a part of a healthy diet. In fact, as previously discussed, nuts are high in monounsaturated and polyunsaturated fats (the "good" fats) as well as plant sterols, all of which have been shown to lower LDL cholesterol.

In 2003, the FDA approved a health claim for seven kinds of nuts stating that "scientific evidence suggests but does not prove that eating 1.5 ounces (45 grams) per day of most nuts as part of a diet low in saturated fat and cholesterol may reduce the risk of heart disease." Instead of simply adding nuts to your diet, the best approach is to eat them in replacement of foods high in saturated fats.

Eat One or Two Meals If You Want to Lose Weight

People who skip meals, especially breakfast, tend to get so hungry that they overeat their next meal or snack to compensate for feeling so hungry. This starts a vicious cycle of bingeing and restricting, which is not only mentally exhausting, but also counterproductive to long-term fat loss. When you skip meals, your metabolism (the rate at which you burn calories) tends to slow down. Eating small meals and snacks (say, three moderate meals and two small snacks) throughout the day helps people control their appetites and their weight.

Don't Eat After 8 P.M. If You Want to Lose Weight

Have you ever been to Spain or France or another European country? If so, you probably noticed that they tend to eat their dinner meal very late compared to the typical American. And, yet, they stay slim. What is going on here?

First, each of us is allotted a certain number of calories to be consumed in a 24-hour time span. Your body does not care when those calories are consumed. Let's say that you are driving down the highway at two in the morning and you notice that your car's gas meter is on empty. You are not going to say, "I can't fill up my gas tank because it's after 8 P.M.," are you? Of course not.

The problem with most Americans is not eating after 8 P.M. It is that most *overeat* after 8 P.M.

The following is the typical American eating profile:

- 6:00 A.M.—out of bed, off to work/school, no breakfast consumed
- 7–8 A.M.—grab coffee on the go
- 10 A.M.—maybe another coffee
- 12 P.M.—small salad, Diet Coke for lunch
- 4 P.M.—gummy bears, Diet Coke from vending machine.
- 6 P.M.—General Tso's Chicken and rice from Chinese restaurant
- 8 P.M.—watch television and snack from a bag of chips
- 11 P.M.—A small bowl of ice cream while watching nightly news
- 12 A.M.—finish off leftover General Tso's chicken and rice and wash it down with some soda before bed

When the person wakes up five to six hours later, they are not hungry for breakfast, so it is skipped (again). But, why would they be after eating so much not so long ago? And then the cycle starts all over again for another day.

It does not matter what time of day you eat. It is what and how much you eat, as well as how much physical activity you do during a 24-hour time span that determines whether you gain, lose, or maintain weight. No matter when you eat, if you do not use all the calories that you have consumed, your body will store the extra calories as fat. Keep in mind that it is a good idea to consume the bulk of your calories during the time of day that you are most active. This way, you not only have plenty of fuel for the tasks at hand, but also are less likely to overeat in the evening.

I'm Skinny, So I Can Eat Whatever I Want

Recall the previous discussion of the "skinny fat person." We now know that being "skinny" or "thin" does not guarantee that you are lean. A skinny-fat person, sometimes referred to as "thin outside, fat inside" (TOFI), typically has very little lean muscle mass and a lot of adipose tissue, which makes their total body weight appear normal.

In fact, fat, active people, sometimes called "fit and fat," can be healthier than their skinny, sedentary counterparts. Normal weight people who are sedentary and unfit are at much higher risk for developing disease than obese persons who are active and fit. How can this be?

Obesity researchers believe that people who are not overweight but still have a high percentage of body fat may have more inflammation in their bodies. These people are often referred to as "normal-weight obese" because of their high body fat percentage.

Chronically high levels of inflammation have been associated with a host of health problems, including heart disease, stroke, hypertension and arthritis.

In reality, a skinny fat person may have a "normal" weight, but this does not make them immune to diabetes or other risk factors for heart disease.

If you are trying to maintain or even lose weight, a healthy diet and exercise can help you increase your lean tissue (muscle) while decreasing your fat stores. This will help increase your metabolism, which will help you burn calories at a quicker rate. Regular physical activity and a healthy diet can help you strengthen your lungs and blood vessels, which can prevent or prolong heart disease. Physical activity and a healthy diet can also improve your blood cholesterol level.

I'm Pregnant, So I'm 'Eating for Two'

The idea that pregnancy is a food free-for-all is a nutrition myth. It is generally recommended that pregnant women increase their daily intake by 100 calories in the first trimester, which is less than one can of Coke! During the second and third trimesters, a pregnant woman should consume 300 extra calories per day.

Being pregnant is not a license to consume whatever you want. The quality of calories consumed is important to ensure the mother's health and the baby's growth and development. Moms-to-be should choose nutrient-rich foods like whole grains, low-fat dairy products, legumes, fruits, and vegetables, which are high in essential nutrients compared to their calorie count.

A daily prenatal multivitamin supplement is often recommended during pregnancy, but you should always talk with your doctor before taking any vitamin or mineral supplements.

Coffee Can Help You Lose Weight

Although coffee and other caffeine products like soda, tea and red bull may temporarily squelch your appetite, drinking a couple of cups a day will not have enough of an effect to help you lose weight. Drinking four to seven cups a day may lead to anxiety, sleeplessness, and an increase in heart rate and blood pressure.

Enjoy a cup or two of coffee every day, but remember that anything added like cream, sugar, or syrup will also add calories. For example, a 16-ounce Starbucks café mocha can contain a whopping 330 calories (60 calories more than some chocolate bars).

Another caffeine concern is sleep disruption, which new evidence reveals is linked to weight control. People become addicted to caffeine especially when sleep deprived, and it takes four to six hours to clear out of your body's system. Drinking caffeine is a quick fix because it only energizes you for 20 to 40 minutes and then you crash. After you crash, your body craves more caffeine or sugar to boost the energy. Now you are setting the stage for a sugar/caffeine roller coaster, which increases your appetite and promotes fat storage. At least two studies have shown that when people are sleep-deprived, they produce more of the hormone ghrelin, an appetite stimulant, and less leptin, an appetite suppressant.

Going on a Diet Is the Best Way to Lose Weight

The first three letters of the word diet (**die**) should give you an indication of how **die**ts fail and make you feel miserable. In the short term, you do lose weight on any plan that results in your eating fewer calories. But temporary changes do not lead to permanent losses.

If you subsist on less than 1,200 calories a day, you will take off weight, but it will not be for long. Consider an analysis of 31 studies of long-term diets, where the diets averaged 1,200 calories a day. The report, published in *American Psychologist,* found that within four to five years, the majority of dieters in these studies regained the weight they had lost. Psychologically, it is difficult for people to adhere to strict diets over a long time period because they feel deprived and hungry. In addition, people who are put on a very-low-calorie diet (800 calories a day) have an increased risk of developing gallstones and digestive issues and their metabolism slows down, which will impair future weight loss.

Do not go on a diet. Instead, change the way you eat. Find a satisfying eating plan that you can live with long term, and make sure you are eating the right amount of calories for weight loss.

But what is the right number of calories for you? Use this easy formula, a favorite of cardiologist Thomas Lee, editor in chief of the *Harvard Heart Letter.*

First find your activity level on the table below. Multiply your weight by the number indicated. (You may fall between two categories. If that is the case, adjust the number by adding a point or so.) The result is the number of calories you need to maintain your weight. Let's say that you weigh 135 pounds and do light exercise one to three days a week. Multiply 135 by 13.5 to get, approximately, 1,800 calories. If you want to drop some pounds, try cutting out 250 calories a day. In a year, if you make no other changes, you could be 26 pounds lighter.

If you. . .

You Exercise: Almost never
Multiply Your Current Weight By: 12

You Exercise: Lightly, one to three days a week
Multiply Your Current Weight By: 13.5

You Exercise: Moderately, three to five days a week
Multiply Your Current Weight By: 15.5

You Exercise: Vigorously, six to seven days a week
Multiply Your Current Weight By: 17

You Exercise: Vigorously, daily, and you have a physical job
Multiply Your Current Weight By: 19

One of the most important aspects of weight maintenance is a high dose of physical activity. The National Weight Control Registry has followed and analyzed the habits of successful weight losers (defined as people who have maintained at least a 30-pound weight loss for a year or more). Among its findings was those who kept weight off exercised with brisk walking, or some other moderate-intensity activity, an average of one hour a day.

Eating Protein and Carbohydrates at Different Meals Will Help You Lose Weight

Your digestive tract can handle a variety of food groups at the same time. There is no proof that eating protein and carbohydrates separately aids digestion or weight loss. Most dietitians agree that it is healthier to combine protein and fiber-filled carbohydrates than to separate them. The pairing of protein and fiber is what fills you up the most and gives you the most energy. An apple is good, but an apple with peanut butter is more filling and controls your blood sugar better.

Eat protein along with carbs, but choose those that are lower in fat. The best protein choices are lean meats, poultry, low-fat dairy products, and tofu. The best carbohydrates are whole grains, fruits, and vegetables. When combined, these foods take longer to absorb, so there is a slower release into the body and a more steady energy source.

ASSIGNMENT #9

Name: _____

Date: _____

1. Interview a family member or friend and quiz them over the above 10 nutrition myths. List which ones they got right or wrong. Be sure to explain the correct answer to those that they got incorrect.

_____
_____
_____
_____
_____
_____
_____
_____
_____
_____
_____
_____
_____
_____
_____
_____
_____
_____
_____
_____
_____
_____

2. Which myths from this chapter were you most surprised to learn? List them. Describe below how you will do things differently in the future related to that myth.

_____
_____
_____
_____
_____
_____
_____
_____
_____
_____
_____
_____
_____
_____
_____
_____
_____
_____
_____
_____
_____

3. Describe why you think people believe nutritional myths?

_____
_____
_____
_____
_____
_____
_____
_____
_____
_____
_____
_____
_____
_____
_____
_____

4. Do you think you know a nutritional myth? What is it and where did you learn about it?

_____

_____

_____

_____

_____

_____

_____

_____

_____

_____

_____

_____

_____

_____

_____

_____

_____

_____

_____

_____

_____

_____

RESOURCES

Ferrier L. K., Caston L. J., Leeson S., Squires J., Weaver B. J., Holub B. J. (1995). Alpha-linolenic acid- and docosahexanaenoic acid-enriched eggs from hens fed flaxseed: influence on blood lipids and platelet phospholipid fatty acids in humans. *American Journal of Clinical Nutrition* 62:81–86.

Ginsberg, H. N., Karmally, W., Siddiqui, M., Holleran, S., Tall, A. R., Blaner, W. S., Ramakrishnan, R. (1995). Increases in dietary cholesterol are associated with modest increases in both LDL and HDL cholesterol in healthy young women. *Arteriosclerosis, Thrombosis, and Vascular Biology* 15:169–178.

Knopp, R. H., Retzlaff, B. M., Walden, C. E., Dowdy, A. A., Tsunehara, C. H. Austin, M. A., Nguyen, T. (1997). A double-blind, randomized trial of the effects of two eggs per day in moderately hypercholesterolemic and combined hyperlipidemic subjects consuming the NCEP Step I diet. *Journal of the American College of Nutrition*, Vol 16, Issue 6: 551–561.

Nestle, Marion. September 24, 2008: The Facts About Corn Sweetner. *San Francisco Chronicle:* http://sfgate.com/cgi-bin/article.cgi?f=/c/a/2008/09/24/FDDS12UH12.DTL This article appeared on page F-1.

United States Department of Agriculture (USDA): www.usda.gov.

EATING BETTER IN AMERICA: PUTTING IT ALL TOGETHER!

Despite efforts to deal with increasingly sedentary lifestyles, Americans are, for the most part, getting fatter. Today, 65 percent of American adults over age 20 are overweight or obese, which is a pretty scary statistic. Just look around and you will realize that you are not alone in needing to learn how to eat better. A cost of $250 billion a year is estimated for medical treatment and lost productivity from obesity and increased risk for heart disease, stroke, high blood pressure, and some forms of cancer. Obesity in our children and teens is of special concern, because an estimated one of every five kids in America today is overweight. Time spent watching television, playing video games, or sitting at the computer contributes to the problem, as do the cutbacks in physical education programs at many schools.

How Did So Many People Get So Heavy?

Most of us are eating more calories than we are burning. The problem of an overweight population comes from a combination of factors:

- Increasing portion sizes,
- More processed foods with fewer nutrients, and
- A more sedentary lifestyle.

We are eating more food. Portions have increased dramatically in the last 20 years. Bigger portions mean that we have to work a lot harder to burn the extra calories that those larger portions add.

We are eating a lot of foods that do not provide many nutrients. We are also consuming more added sugars, which is found in carbonated drinks, fruit drinks, sports beverages, and processed foods. Evidence suggests that drinking calorie-containing beverages may not make you feel full, which can lead you to eat and drink more than you need, adding even more calories to your diet.

We are eating out more often than ever before. The danger in eating out is that many types of food eaten away from home, including fast-food and prepared meals you buy at the grocery store are high in saturated fat, trans fat, cholesterol, added sugars and sodium. They also can be low in fiber and vitamins and minerals. In addition, people tend to eat larger portions when eating out.

We are less active. Current estimates indicate that more than half of the adults in the United States do not engage in any regular physical activity at all. As we spend more of our free time in front of televisions, computers and video games, we are more likely to put on pounds. Our increasingly sedentary lifestyles are putting us at risk for serious health problems, including cardiovascular disease, type 2 diabetes, osteoporosis, depression, and breast and colon cancer.

What Eating Healthier Will Do for You

Eating healthy food will help you to:

- Feel great and have energy to enjoy life more
- Have a strong immune system so you stay well, even when everyone else is getting sick
- Maintain a healthy weight and look physically fit
- Stay as alert and mentally sharp at 60, 70, and even 80 as you were at 20
- Do the same things at 65 that you did at 20, with the same gusto
- Live to be 100, and be physically fit and active
- Prevent certain diseases known to be a related to diet and nutrition, particularly cancer, heart disease, stroke, high blood pressure, high cholesterol, diabetes and obesity

Some of the things that you could experience if you are not eating healthfully might include:

- Headaches
- Indigestion
- Depression
- Candida yeast
- Difficulty sleeping
- Poor memory
- Senile dementia
- Anorexia and bulimia
- Dry skin
- Adult acne
- Constipation
- Poor digestion
- Halitosis (bad breath)
- Mouth and tongue ulcers
- Menstrual problems
- Diarrhea
- Irritability
- Fatigue
- Polyps
- Diverticulitis
- Gallstones
- Osteoporosis
- COPD—(chronic obstructive pulmonary disease)
- Anemia
- Asthma
- Mental illness
- Irritable bowel syndrome
- Fibromyalgia

Our fast-food culture is one where meals have become yet another task that we squeeze in during the day. American adults devote an average of 1 hour and 12 minutes per day to eating, yet spend between 2 and 3 hours per day watching television. American youth kids are rushed too. Studies have shown that school lunch periods provide an average of 7 to 11 minutes for students to consume their lunch.

Healthy eating is not about strict dieting, staying unrealistically thin, or depriving yourself of the foods you love; instead it is about feeling great, having more energy, and keeping yourself as healthy as possible.

When you want to lose weight, is your first choice to run to the latest fad diet? Often a quick 5 to 10 pounds will come off, then your old eating habits return and you end up gaining more weight and slowing downing you metabolism. Preoccupation with body shape, size, and weight creates an unhealthy lifestyle of emotional and physical deprivation.

Decades of research have shown that diets, both self-initiated and professionally led, are ineffective at producing long-term health and weight loss or weight control. Only 5 percent of people who go on diets are successful; 95 percent of all traditional diets fail. When you go on a low-calorie diet, your body thinks you are starving. It actually becomes more efficient at storing fat by slowing down your metabolism. When you stop dieting, your metabolism is still slow and inefficient and you gain the weight back even faster. In addition, low-calorie diets cause you to lose both muscle and fat in equal amounts. However, when you eventually gain back the weight, it is all fat and not muscle, causing your metabolism to slow down even more.

Staying healthy is a life-long proposition. Do not waste your time, energy, and money on "quick fix" solutions. Fad diets, diet pills, protein powders, liposuction, and even intestinal or gastric bypass surgery might provide a leaner profile, but they do not provide the nutrients needed to keep you as healthy as you could be.

You should also consider that most diets are a temporary fix and may not result in your goal of long-term weight loss. As you consider each of these diets, note the number of calories it allows.

Comparison of Calories Among Major Diet Books

Book	Calories	Calorie Source	Claims	Points to Consider
Eat More, Weigh Less by Dean Ornish, MD	1,500	80% carbohydrates (CHO), 15% proteins, 5% fat, 40 g fiber	Fat free is key to weight loss.	Without a dietician's help, hard to maintain with so little fat. Fat provides flavor and texture to our food.
Sugar Busters by Steward, Andrews, and Balart	1,600	35% CHO, 25% proteins, 40% fat, 20 g fiber	Refined CHO cause weight gain by raising blood sugar.	There is no scientific evidence to support this claim.
Dr. Atkins' Diet Revolution by Robert Atkins, MD	1,800	15% CHO, 30% proteins, 55% fat, 10g fiber	Only CHO make you fat. Eliminate them and your body burns fat.	There is no scientific evidence to support this claim. If you eliminate some calories, no matter what the source, your body must find energy elsewhere.

continues

Comparison of Calories Among Major Diet Books (*Continued*)

Book	Calories	Calorie Source	Claims	Points to Consider
Protein Power by Michael and Mary Dan Eades	1,700	15% CHO, 25% proteins, 60% fat, 50 g fiber	Limits CHO lowers insulin and insulin causes obesity.	This claim has been refuted by scientific research. It would be hard to maintain on this diet because CHOs are ubiquitous. We also know that a diet with 60% fat will increase your risk for heart disease. The diet does not allow for individual variation.
The Zone by Barry Sears	1,000	40% CHO, 30% proteins, 30% fat, 50 g fiber	Claims the FDA 60:15:30 ratio of CHO, protein, and fats causes weight gain. Changing to his 40:30:30 plan will result in weight loss.	The ratio is not the problem; the number of calories is the problem!
Dieting with the Duchess by Weight Watchers	1,400	55% CHO, 25% proteins, 20% fats, 25 g fiber	Food choices based on point system. Eat only the required points, you lose weight.	An easy to maintain calorie reduction method, with appropriate choices. This has been shown to produce long-term success.
The South Beach Diet by Arthur Agatston, MD	No calorie count is specified, but calories are greatly reduced in the first 2 weeks by eliminating CHO and fruit.	Emphasizes healthy fats and allows only low glycemic index CHO. No bread, potatoes, fruits, corn, carrots, rice, or cereal in first 2 weeks and strongly discouraged even after the initiation phase.	Claims foods that are high on the glycemic index result in more weight gain.	The diet restricts many healthful food choices. There is no science to support that these high glycemic index foods lead to more weight gain. Exercise is not promoted.

Healthy eating is not just what you eat, but how you eat. Paying attention to what you eat and choosing foods that are both nourishing and enjoyable helps support an overall healthy diet. A better plan for healthy eating is one that is comprised of nutrient dense calories from all the essential food groups together with an exercise plan to which you can adhere. However, even this new healthy eating plan will not work unless you become responsible for what you eat, responsible for exercising, and accountable when you relapse. If you do relapse, just remember the days when you were successful and get back on track.

- Take time to chew your food. Chew your food slowly, savoring every bite. We tend to rush though our meals, forgetting to actually taste the flavors and feel the textures of what is in our mouths.
- Avoid eating while stress. When we are stressed, our digestion can be compromised, causing problems like colitis and heartburn. Avoid eating while working, driving, arguing, or watching television. Try taking some deep breaths before beginning your meal.
- Stop multitasking. We often pair eating with other activities, such as driving or working at our desks. Eating while multitasking, whether working through lunch or watching television while eating dinner, often leads us to eat more.

- Listen to your body. Ask yourself if you are really hungry, and stop eating when you feel full. It actually takes a few minutes for your brain to tell your body that it has had enough food, so eat slowly.
- Eat mindfully. Eating mindfully means eating with awareness—not awareness of what foods are on your plate, but rather awareness of the experience of eating. Mindful eating is being present, moment by moment, for each sensation that happens during eating, such as chewing, tasting and swallowing. Mindless eating, or eating without awareness, can have negative health consequences. It turns out that when our mind is tuned out during mealtime, the digestive process may be 30 percent to 40 percent less effective, which can contribute to digestive distress, such as gas, bloating and bowel irregularities, overeating and obesity.

How to Practice Eating Mindfully

Mindful eating means paying attention to what you eat and savoring each bite. Being mindful also means noticing when you are almost full and laying down your fork. Mindful eating relaxes you so you digest better and makes you feel more satisfied.

Eat with awareness of the taste, chew, bite, or swallow. Try the following exercise.

1. Take one bite of an apple slice (or any food) and then close your eyes. Do not begin chewing yet.
2. Try not to pay attention to the ideas running through your mind, just focus on the apple. Notice anything that comes to mind about taste, texture, temperature, and sensation going on in your mouth.
3. Begin chewing now. Chew slowly, just noticing that what it feels like. It is normal that your mind will want to wander off. If you notice that you are paying more attention to your thinking than to the chewing, just let go of the thought for the moment and come back to the chewing. Notice each tiny movement of your jaw.
4. In these moments, you may find yourself wanting to swallow the apple. See if you can stay present and notice the subtle transition from chewing to swallowing.
5. As you prepare to swallow the apple, try to follow it moving toward the back of your tongue and into your throat. Swallow the apple, following it until you can no longer feel any sensation of the food remaining.
6. Take a deep breath and exhale.

Diet Strategies That Work

- Choose foods that contain fewer calories and more fiber, which will fill you up.
- Eating five smaller meals might work better than eating three larger ones. The goal is to eat a small amount of food every 3 hours or so.
- Eat less cholesterol and less fat especially less saturated fat and no trans fat. Fats are very high in calories.
- Eat more fiber to fool your stomach. Reduce the calories by focusing on water-dense fruits and vegetables therefore, you can keep the volume high and feel satisfied. Your stomach senses food volume, it has stretch receptors and pressure sensors. Start meals with a big salad—lots of vegetables with no croutons or creamy dressing like Caesar dressing; have double portions of fruit and vegetables at meals and skip or cut back on calorie-dense starches, fats, and fatty meats. Opt for a fruit dessert, with a dab of sorbet for flavor.
- Eat quality carbohydrates. Choosing low-glycemic foods like fruits, vegetables, and whole grains over refined foods (e.g., sodas, doughnuts, white potatoes) could help keep you from gaining 10 extra pounds even if you do not cut calories. Low-glycemic eating makes blood sugar stay lower, you feel full faster, and the body does not seem to react to the diet with as much stress.

- Choose whole grain cereal, pasta, rice, and bread. Many foods that claim they are "whole wheat" or "whole grain" on the front of the package are really made with mostly white, processed flour, which is not nearly as nutritious. Always check the ingredients to see if "whole wheat" or "whole grain" is the first ingredient listed; do not be fooled by how a food looks. For example, some dark brown breads are colored with coffee or other dyes, not whole grains.
- Avoid food that is high in sugar, like pastries, sweetened cereal, and soda or fruit-flavored drinks.
- Watch what you drink.

Beverage	Calories/16 Ounces
Ice cream milk shakes	538
Grape juice	307
Orange juice	224
Cola	200
Iced teas, sugared	200
Beer	195
Sports drinks	100
Water	0

- Reduced-fat or no-fat (skim) milk, reduced-fat cheese, and low-fat or no-fat yogurt are good sources of needed protein and calcium.
- Exercise more to burn calories. Research has shown that 30 minutes of moderately strenuous daily exercise is also one of the most important requirements for disease prevention—even for people who are already at an ideal weight. For example what 3,400 more steps a day for 3 months will do the following for you:

3.3 pounds loss

0.6-point reduction in BMI

1-centimeter drop in waist circumference

4-beat-per-minute drop in resting heart rate

11,550 extra calories burned

- Eat nuts. The protein, fat, and fiber in almonds keep you feeling full. Have a handful (no more they are also high in calories) in place of your usual midmorning or after-noon snack.
- Let the sun in. A host of solid new studies from leading institutions link light deprivation to a wide variety of weight-related disorders including depression, bulimia, and PMS. People who are chronically deprived of light exposure can have profound effects on dietary choices, energy levels, physical activity, and weight gain. Susceptible people experience overwhelming food cravings, lethargy, and weight gain (some more than 30 pounds) during dark winter months.
- Get a good night's sleep. Lack of sleep may pack on extra pounds. In a recent study at the University of Chicago, people who slept only 4 hours a night for 2 nights had a 28% higher level of ghrelin (the eat-more hormone) and an 18% lower level of leptin (the eat-less hormone) than those who slept more. (Ann of Int Med, 2004).

To manage your weight safely and for the long term, You should plan meals and snacks throughout the day.

The major components of a successful, life-long weight management plan are:

1. Recognizing you have control over what you eat,

2. Recognizing that you can choose to make time to exercise,

3. Ensuring that the calories you consume are equal to the calories you spend if you want to stay the same weight.

4. Ensuring that the calories you consume are less than the calories you spend if you want to lose weight.

5. Ensuring that the calories you consume are more than the calories you spend if you want to gain weight.

HEALTHIER GROCERY SHOPPING

To be a healthier grocery shopper, spend more time in the outer aisles of the store where fresh foods are kept. Spend less time in the middle aisles where packaged foods, snacks, and soft drinks are stocked.

Shopping List

- Fresh vegetables and fruits should make up the largest part of your healthy foods grocery list.
- Purchase grain and cereal products made from whole grains, not from refined flours. This part of your list includes whole grain breads, whole grain pastas, and whole grain breakfast cereals. Whole grains are important for vitamins, minerals, and for fiber, which is often lacking in modern diets. Read labels to look for 100 percent whole grain or 100 percent whole wheat to ensure you are getting whole grain products.
- Your protein and meat choices should consist mostly of fish, poultry and lean meats. Eggs, nuts, seeds and legumes are also good sources of protein. Choose fresh and frozen unbreaded meats and fish. Avoid breaded, deep-fried convenience foods that you put in the oven. They are high in fats and sodium.
- Beverages should be kept simple. Water, low-fat milk, juices, and herbal teas are all good choices. If you choose soft drinks, choose diet ones to avoid extra sugar.
- Dairy products should include low-fat milk, yogurt and cheese. If you do not want cows' milk, choose soy and rice beverages, calcium fortified orange juice, or goats' milk and cheese.
- Be careful with dressings, cooking oils, and condiments. They are sneaky sources of refined sugar and poor quality oils. Read labels to choose dressings made with olive oil, canola oil or walnut oil. Choose low-fat mayonnaise for your sandwiches, and choose canola oil and olive oil for cooking.
- Frozen foods are a convenient way to keep vegetables on hand. Prepared meals that you can pop into the microwave or oven can be convenient and healthy if you choose low-fat versions with good portion sizes. Read labels and chose frozen foods wisely. Avoid frozen pizzas, pocket-sandwiches, deep-fried appetizers, and breaded foods.
- Foods in cans and jars are also very convenient. Look for low-sodium soups, vegetables, and sauces. Avoid high-fat gravies and high-calorie foods like canned spaghetti and ravioli products.
- For sandwiches, choose peanut butter or other nut butters, low-fat turkey slices, or sliced roast beef. Avoid processed lunch meats, sausages, and hot dogs.
- Do not load up on high calorie treats and desserts. Choose fresh fruits, healthy nuts, seeds, and whole grain crackers for snacks.

Reading Food Labels

When you go grocery shopping, take time to read the nutrition labels on your purchases. Compare nutrients and calories in one food to those in another. Pay attention to the serving size and the

Product: **Check for:**

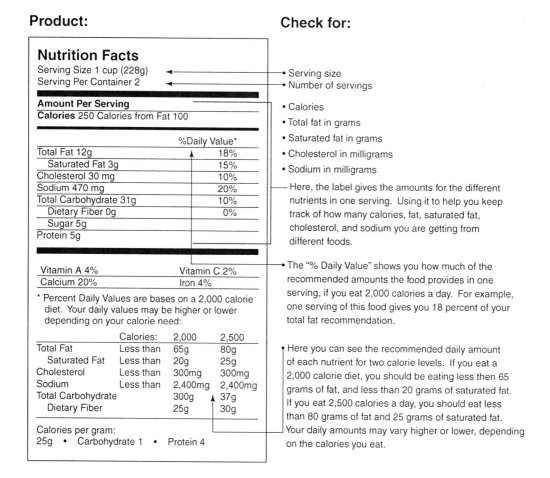

- Serving size
- Number of servings
- Calories
- Total fat in grams
- Saturated fat in grams
- Cholesterol in milligrams
- Sodium in milligrams

Here, the label gives the amounts for the different nutrients in one serving. Using it to help you keep track of how many calories, fat, saturated fat, cholesterol, and sodium you are getting from different foods.

The "% Daily Value" shows you how much of the recommended amounts the food provides in one serving, if you eat 2,000 calories a day. For example, one serving of this food gives you 18 percent of your total fat recommendation.

Here you can see the recommended daily amount of each nutrient for two calorie levels. If you eat a 2,000 calorie diet, you should be eating less then 65 grams of fat, and less than 20 grams of saturated fat. If you eat 2,500 calories a day, you should eat less than 80 grams of fat and 25 grams of saturated fat. Your daily amounts may vary higher or lower, depending on the calories you eat.

servings per container. All labels list total calories in a serving size of the product. Compare the total calories in the product that you choose with others like it; choose the one that is lowest in calories.

The "Nutrition Facts" label contains this information:

Serving size: If you eat double the serving size listed, you need to double the calories, fat, and nutrients. If you eat half the size shown, cut the calories and nutrients in half.

Calories: This is very helpful to know if you're cutting calories to lose weight.

Total Fat: The label gives you the number of grams of fat per serving (so you can track your daily intake) and the number of calories from fat. If you are overweight or trying to lose weight, you should set a goal of an overall intake of no more than 25 to 35 percent of your total calories from fat, with less than 7 percent as saturated fat and less than 1 percent as trans fat.

Saturated fat: It is a key nutrient for raising your blood cholesterol and your risk of heart disease and stroke. Eat less saturated fat!

Cholesterol: Too much cholesterol in your diet may lead to too much of it in your blood. Too much cholesterol in your blood can lead to heart disease and stroke. It is best to eat less than 300 mg each day. People with heart disease, high LDL cholesterol levels or who are taking cholesterol medication should consume less than 200 mg of cholesterol per day.

Sodium: Watch for both natural and added sodium. Ordinary table salt is sodium chloride, 40 percent sodium by weight. Healthy adults should take in less than 2,300 mg of sodium each day, which is equal to about 1 teaspoon of salt. African-Americans, middle-aged and older adults, and people with high blood pressure need less than 1,500 mg per day.

Total Carbohydrate: Emphasize fruits, vegetables, and whole-grain breads and cereals.

Dietary Fiber: Fruits, vegetables, whole grains, peas, and beans are good sources and can help reduce the risk of heart disease.

Protein: Most animal protein contains fat and cholesterol, therefore eat small portions.

Vitamins and Minerals: Eating a variety of foods will help you reach your daily goal of 100 percent of vitamin A, vitamin C, calcium and iron.

Daily Value: The daily values are guides for people who eat 2,000 calories each day. If you eat more or less than that, your daily value may be higher or lower. Choose foods with a low percent daily value of fat, saturated fat, cholesterol, and sodium. Try to reach 100 percent of the daily value of total carbohydrates, dietary fiber, vitamins, and minerals.

EATING HEALTHY ON A BUDGET

Today Americans are paying at the gas pump but also and at the grocery store. Preparing your own food is one of the best ways to make sure that you are making healthy choices. It is also a great way to save money compared to eating out or buying prepared meals. Eating healthier foods can actually save you money. According to a 2002 study published in the *Journal of the American Dietetic Association,* the researchers found that when families went on weight loss diets, they not only lost weight but also reduced their food budgets. The savings came from reducing portion sizes and from buying fewer of the high-calorie foods that tend to increase the amount spent at the grocery store (Glanz et al., 1998). People tend to spend a lot on those "extras," foods that add calories but little nutritional value, like sodas, bakery items, and chips. The ideal food is nutrient-dense, not calorie-dense, and the least expensive may be fresh, frozen, or canned. Save money by passing on calorie-dense cakes and cookies; instead, opt for seasonal fruit.

Tips for Eating Healthy on a Budget

- Have a light snack before you go grocery shopping, and stick to your grocery list to help avoid impulse purchases or costly mistakes like falling for the displays at the end of the aisles.
- Before you plan your weekly menu, check the ads to see what is on sale and use money-saving coupons.
- Check the food section in your newspaper to find the best buys for the week, based on fresh produce in season. Shop your local farmers' market for great deals on local produce.
- Planning meals around what is on sale can lower your grocery bills, especially if you also use coupons. Stock up on staples when they are on sale.
- Making lunch and taking it with you is a great money-saver and an excellent use of leftovers. Packing your lunch not only saves you money, but also allows you control all the ingredients so they are healthy and low in calories.
- Using frozen foods may be less expensive than fresh, yet they are equally nutritious. Produce is typically frozen at the peak of ripeness, when nutrients are plentiful. Fish and poultry are often flash-frozen to minimize freezer damage and retain freshness. With frozen foods, you can use only the amount you need, reseal the package, and return it to the freezer.
- Substitute inexpensive, vegetarian sources such as beans, eggs, tofu, and legumes for more expensive meat, fish, or poultry. Eat vegetarian once a week or more to increase your consumption of healthy plant foods while saving money. Eggs are an excellent, inexpensive source of protein that can be eaten for breakfast, lunch or dinner.
- Go generic. Consider buying store brands instead of pricier national brands. Read the ingredient list on the label to be sure that you are getting the most for your money.

- Try to concentrate your shopping around the outer aisles of the store and avoid the inner aisles. The outer aisles tend to house the fresh vegetables, meats, eggs and dairy products. The inner aisles tend to contain mostly processed foods, which are more expensive and less healthy.
- If you head to the grocery store when you are hungry, you are more likely to give into impulse and buy expensive, unhealthy junk food. Have a healthy snack, like a piece of fruit or a quick salad, before you head out.

HEALTHY EATING OUT

Americans are eating out more than ever. When dining out, it is easy to eat more calories and fat as well as food that is less healthy.

Tips for Healthy Eating Out

- Practice eating small portions. At a typical restaurant, a single serving provides enough for two meals. Take half the entrée home or split the meal with a friend. Order an appetizer as a main course instead.
- Go to places where you can order healthy, low-fat meals.
- According to the Center for Science in the Public Interest, soft drinks are the single biggest source of calories in the American diet. One 32 ounce Big Gulp with non-diet cola packs about 425 calories, so one Big Gulp can quickly gulp up a big portion of your daily calorie intake. Try switching to water with lemon or unsweetened iced tea.
- Request items be made without butter or oil. Ask for your vegetables and main dishes to be served without the sauces. If your food is fried or cooked in oil or butter, ask to have it broiled or steamed. Ask to substitute high-fat items like french fries for a baked potato or side salad instead.
- Eat a little less at noon to save for a special dinner later, but do not skip meals which can lead to eating too much.
- Eat something 30 minutes before your meal to help be in better control of your choices. Eat a piece of fruit or have a glass of water with lemon.
- Avoid buffets, and all-you-can-eat specials. You will likely overeat to get your money's worth. If you do choose buffet dining, opt for fresh fruits, salads with low-fat dressings, broiled entrees and steamed vegetables. Resist the temptation to go for seconds, or wait at least 20 minutes after eating to make sure that you are really still hungry before going back up to the buffet.
- Dishes labeled "deep-fried," "pan-fried," "basted," "batter-dipped," "breaded, creamy," "crispy," "scalloped," "Alfredo," "au gratin," or "in cream sauce" are usually high in calories, unhealthy fats, or sodium.
- Be aware of calorie- and fat-packed salad dressings, spreads, cheese, and sour cream. For example, ask for a grilled chicken sandwich without the mayonnaise.
- Breaded, batter-dipped, and tempura all are fried food, which is heavy in fat. Look instead for lower fat, grilled, broiled and flame-cooked. Other good choices include entrees that are steamed, poached, roasted, or baked in their own juices.
- For sauces, stick to wine, or thinned, stock-based sauces. Avoid thick butter sauces, béarnaise, Mornay or sauces that sound creamy.
- If ordering pizza, ask for extra vegetable toppings and forget the meats and extra cheese.
- Count alcohol calories as part of your eating. Alcohol is very high in calories and can prevent us from making healthy food choices.

What to Order When Eating Out

Fast Food

Be aware that the average fast-food meal can easily run more than 1,000 calories and contain a full day's worth of sodium. Check the nutritional value of foods by asking the restaurant or checking the restaurant's website before you go. Choose the salads, water or diet sodas or the children's portion if you are craving that food. Also, if you eat fast food for one meal, plan around it to cut the rest of the day's calories, sodium, and sugars and increase fruits and vegetables.

- Watch out for word like jumbo, giant, deluxe, biggie-sized or super-sized. Larger portions mean extra calories and more fat, cholesterol, sodium, and sugar.
- Avoid eating croissants and biscuits because they have lots of extra fat and very little fiber.
- End a meal with sugar-free, fat-free yogurt. Ices, sorbets, and sherbets have less fat, but still have lots of sugar. Bring a piece of fruit from home for your dessert after eating lunch out.
- Be alert for tricky information. For example, a fat-free muffin is fat free but much higher in sugar than another muffin. Chinese food may seem okay if you order steamed vegetables, but if you use lots of soy sauce you get too much sodium.
- Choose barbequed or broiled and grilled chicken sandwiches—as well as a regular hamburger or roast beef sandwich—instead of jumbo burgers and fried sandwiches.

EATING OUT: HEALTHY AND UNHEALTHY CHOICES

Burger Chains

Healthy Choices	Unhealthy Choices
Regular, single-patty hamburger without mayonnaise or cheese	Double-patty hamburger with cheese, mayonnaise, special sauce, and bacon
Grilled chicken sandwich	Fried chicken sandwich
Veggie burger	Fried fish sandwich
Garden salad with grilled chicken and low-fat dressing	Salad with toppings such as bacon, cheese, and ranch dressing
Egg on a muffin	Breakfast burrito with steak
Baked potato	French fries
Yogurt parfait	Milk shake
Grilled chicken strips	Chicken "nuggets" or tenders
Limiting cheese, mayonnaise, and special sauces	Adding cheese, extra mayonnaise, and special sauces

Fried Chicken Chains

Healthy Choices	Unhealthy Choices
Skinless chicken breast without breading	Fried chicken (original or extra-crispy)
Honey barbeque chicken sandwich	Teriyaki wings or popcorn chicken
Garden salad	Caesar salad
Mashed potatoes	Chicken and biscuit "bowl"
Limiting gravy and sauces	Adding extra gravy and sauces

Taco Chains

Healthy Choices	Unhealthy Choices
Grilled chicken soft taco	Crispy shell chicken taco
Black beans	Refried beans
Shrimp ensalada	Steak chalupa
Grilled "fresco" style steak burrito	Crunch wraps or gordita-type burritos
Vegetable and bean burrito	Nachos with refried beans
Limiting sour cream, guacamole, or cheese	Adding sour cream, guacamole, or cheese

Subs, Sandwich and Deli Choices

Healthy Choices	Unhealthy Choices
Six-inch sub	Foot-long sub
Lean meat (roast beef, chicken breast, lean ham) or vegetables	High-fat meat such as ham, tuna salad, bacon, meatballs, or steak
One or two slices of lower-fat cheese (Swiss or mozzarella)	The "normal" amount of higher-fat (Cheddar, American) cheese
Adding low-fat dressing or mustard instead of mayo	Adding mayonnaise and special sauces
Adding extra vegetable toppings	Keeping the sub "as is" with all toppings
Choosing whole-grain bread or taking the top slice off your sub and eating it open-faced	Choosing white bread or "wraps" which are often higher in fat than normal

Casual-fare Restaurant Choices

Healthy Choices	Unhealthy Choices
Side salad with low-fat dressing or a side of steamed vegetables	Salads with fried onions, cheeses, meats and high-fat dressings
Turkey, roast beef, or grilled chicken sandwich	Mayonnaise-heavy tuna or chicken salad sandwich
Baked or grilled fish	Battered or deep-fried fish
Chicken or turkey wraps without mayonnaise or cheese	Extra-large burgers loaded with cheese and sauces

Asian Food Choices

Healthy Choices	Unhealthy Choices
Egg drop, miso, wonton, or hot and sour soup	Fried egg rolls, spare ribs, tempura
Stir-fried, steamed, roasted, or broiled entrees (shrimp chow mein, chop suey)	Battered or deep-fried dishes (sweet and sour pork, General Tso's chicken)
Steamed or baked tofu	Deep-fried tofu
Sauces such as ponzu, rice-wine vinegar, wasabi, ginger, and low-sodium soy sauce	Coconut milk, sweet and sour sauce, regular soy sauce
Steamed brown rice	Fried rice
Edamame, cucumber salad, stir-fried vegetables	Salads with fried or crispy noodles

Italian and Pizza Restaurant Choices

Healthy Choices	Unhealthy Choices
Thin-crust pizza with half the cheese and extra vegetables	Thick-crust or butter-crust pizza with extra cheese and meat toppings
Plain rolls or breadsticks	Garlic bread
Antipasto with vegetables	Antipasto with meat
Pasta with tomato sauce and vegetables	Pasta with cream or butter-based sauce (Alfredo)
Red sauce (marinara, red clam, or marsala	Entree with side of pasta
Entree with side of vegetables	Fried ("Frito") dishes
Grilled ("Griglia") dishes	Parmigiana, beef lasagna
	Cheese sauce or filling, pesto, carbonara, sausage dishes

Steakhouse

- Trim the fat from broiled meat and order without sauces or gravy.
- A filet, flank, or London broil steak is the leanest cut.

Salad Bar

- Be careful about potato and pasta salads, bacon bits, marinated vegetables, olives, fruits in heavy syrup, and seeds or nuts.
- One ladle of creamy salad dressing can be about 300 calories.
- Select dark, leafy greens, raw vegetables and fruits, lean ham or turkey, and cottage cheese.
- Use fat-free dressing or low-fat dressing in small amounts.

Pizza

- Vegetable pizzas can have half the calories of the "works" type.
- Ask for extra vegetables to replace the meat on pizza.
- You can request half of the cheese as well.

Mexican

- Chicken fajitas, tortillas, and Spanish rice without sour cream and guacamole are often okay choices.
- Go easy on chips and rich or fried items on the menu such as chili rellanos, nachos, chorizo, chimichangas, flautas, and taco bowl salads.

FOOD ADDITIVES

There are more than 3000 different food additives that are purposefully added to our food supply. Some of them are known to cause cancer!

Food additives that are common in most packaged foods can:

- Make you fat
- Give you cancer
- Cause you to get diabetes

- Give you heart disease
- Cause high blood pressure
- Cause hormone imbalances

Food Additive Safety Codes

The following codes indicate the safety of the additives in the table below. Many additives have more than one code used to describe their safety.

*	GRAS—Generally recognized as safe by the FDA
§	FDA-approved colorant
S	There is no known toxicity. The additive appears to be safe.
A	The additive may cause allergic reactions.
C	Caution is advised. The additive may be unsafe, poorly tested, or used in foods eaten often.
C1	Caution is advised for certain groups in the population, such as pregnant women, infants, persons with high blood pressure, and kidney problems.
X	The additive is unsafe or very poorly tested.

Some Common Food Additives

-	X	-	Acesulfame-K: may cause low blood sugar attacks; causes cancer, elevated cholesterol in lab animals
-	X	-	Acesulfame-potassium: same as acesulfame-K
-	C	-	Animal or vegetable shortening: associated with heart disease, hardening of the arteries, and elevated cholesterol levels
-	X	A	Artificial color FD & C, U.S certified food color: contribute to hyperactivity in children; may contribute to learning and visual disorders, nerve damage; may be carcinogenic; see FD&C Colors
-	X	A	Artificial flavoring: may cause reproductive disorders, and developmental problems; not adequately tested
-	X	-	Artificial sweeteners: associated with health problems; see specific sweetener
-	X	-	Aspartame: may cause brain damage in phenylketonurics; may cause central nervous system disturbances, menstrual difficulties; may affect brain development in unborn fetus
*	X	A	BHA: can cause liver and kidney damage, behavioral problems, infertility, weakened immune system, birth defects, cancer; should be avoided by infants, young children, pregnant women, and those sensitive to aspirin
*	X	A	BHT: see BHA; banned in England
-	X	A	Brominated vegetable oil: linked to major organ system damage, birth defects, growth problems; considered unsafe by the FDA, can still lawfully be used unless further action is taken by the FDA
*	X	-	Caffeine: psychoactive, addictive drug; may cause fertility problems, birth defects, heart disease, depression, nervousness, behavioral changes, and insomnia
§	X	-	FD&C Colors: colors considered safe by the FDA for use in food, drugs and cosmetics; most of the colors are derived from coal tar and must be certified by the FDA not to contain more than 10 ppm of lead and arsenic; certification does not address any harmful effects these colors may have on the body; most coal tar colors are potential carcinogens, may contain carcinogenic contaminants, and cause allergic reactions

-	X	-	Free glutamates: may cause brain damage, especially in children; always found in autolyzed yeast, calcium caseinate, enzymes, flavors and flavorings, gelatin, glutamate, glutamic acid, hydrolyzed protein, hydrolyzed soy protein, plant protein extract, protease, protease enzymes, sodium caseinate, textured protein, yeast extract, yeast food and yeast nutrient; may be in barley malt, boullion, broth, carrageenan, malt extract, malt flavoring, maltodextrin, natural flavors, natural chicken flavoring, natural beef flavoring, natural pork flavoring, pectin, seasonings, soy protein, soy protein concentrate, soy protein isolate, soy sauce, soy sauce extract, stock, whey protein, whey protein concentrate, whey protein isolate, anything that is enzyme modified, fermented, protein fortified, or ultrapasteurized and foods that advertise 'NO MSG'; see MSG
-	X	A	Hydrogenated vegetable oil: associated with heart disease, breast and colon cancer, atherosclerosis, elevated cholesterol
	X	A	Hydrolyzed vegetable protein—may cause brain and nervous system damage in infants; high salt content; may be corn, soy, or wheat based; contains free glutamates
*	X	A	MSG: may cause headaches, itching, nausea, brain, nervous system, reproductive disorders, high blood pressure; pregnant, lactating mothers, infants, and small children should avoid; allergic reactions common; may be hidden in infant formula, low-fat milk, candy, chewing gum, drinks, over-the-counter medications, especially children's, binders and fillers for nutritional supplements, prescription and non-prescription drugs, IV fluids given in hospitals, chicken pox vaccine; being sprayed on growing fruits and vegetables as a growth enhancer; proposed for use on organic crops
-	X	A	Natural flavors: may be chemically extracted and processed and in combination with other food additives not required to be listed on the label; may contain free glutamates; see MSG
-	X	-	Nitrates: form powerful cancer-causing agents in stomach; can cause death; considered dangerous by FDA, but not banned because they prevent botulism
-	X	-	Nitrites: may cause headaches, nausea, vomiting, dizziness; see nitrates

Cancer-Causing Ingredients Found in Some Food

BHA is a preservative that the International Agency for Research on Cancer (IARC) classifies as a possible carcinogen; it possibly causes cancer. It may be used to preserve foods, like cereal, that come in a box, or it may be sprayed on the packaging instead. Either way it should be avoided.

Potassium bromate is in brominated flour, often found in bread. It is classified as a possible carcinogen. Most countries in the world have banned this ingredient, except for the United States and Japan.

Citrus Red No. 2, or FD&C Citrus Red No. 2, is also a possible carcinogen. Its use is limited to coloring orange skins. If you eat the orange peel or grate it to use in any foods that you make, you will be eating a chemical that possibly causes cancer.

FD&C Colors are generally derived from coal tar. Coal tar is a human carcinogen. It is known to cause cancer.

Smoked foods may contain nitrosmaines and polycyclic aromatic hydrocarbons (PAH), both of which can cause cancer. There is not enough information to know if smoked flavorings pose the same risk.

Most processed meats, unless you buy organic and nitrite-free, contain nitrates or nitrites, which are chemicals that are classified as probable carcinogens by the IARC. In other words, they probably cause cancer.

Processed Meats Include:

- Bacon
- Ham

- Sausage
- Hot dogs
- Pepperoni
- Salami
- Pastrami
- Bologna
- Deli meats, like chicken, turkey, roast beef
- Pickled vegetables that are prepared the traditional way as done in Asia

MENU PLANNING IS THE KEY

When you take the time to plan out menus, you can creatively use leftovers, buy only the food you need, and save time and money. Meal planning also makes you think about foods that will satisfy your needs.

Sample Menus for a 2,000 Calorie Food Pattern

Breakfast	Lunch	Snacks	Dinner
(Choose one below)	*(Choose one below)*	*(Choose one below)*	*(Choose one below)*
Breakfast burrito	Roast beef sandwich	1 cup cantaloupe	Stuffed broiled salmon
1 flour tortilla (7" diameter)	*1 whole grain sandwich bun*		*5 ounce salmon filet*
1 scrambled egg (in 1 tsp soft margarine)	*3 ounces lean roast beef*		*1 ounce bread stuffing mix*
⅓ cup black beans	*2 slices tomato*		*1 tbsp diced celery*
2 tbsp salsa	*¼ cup shredded romaine lettuce*		*2 tsp canola oil*
1 cup orange juice	*⅛ cup sauteed mushrooms (in 1 tsp oil)*		*½ cup saffron (white) rice*
1 cup fat-free milk	*1 ½ ounce part-skim mozzarella cheese*		*1 ounce slivered almonds*
	1 tsp yellow mustard		*½ cup steamed broccoli*
	¾ cup baked potato wedges		*1 tsp soft margarine*
	1 tbsp ketchup		1 cup fat-free milk
	1 unsweetened beverage		

Breakfast	Lunch	Snacks	Dinner
(Choose one below)	*(Choose one below)*	*(Choose one below)*	*(Choose one below)*
Hot cereal	Taco salad	½ ounce dry-roasted almonds	Spinach lasagna
½ cup cooked oatmeal	*2 ounces tortilla chips*	¼ cup pineapple	*1 cup lasagna noodles, cooked (2 oz dry)*
2 tbsp raisins	*2 ounces ground turkey, sauteed in 2 tsp sunflower oil*	2 tbsp raisins	*⅔ cup cooked spinach*
1 tsp soft margarine	*½ cup black beans*		*½ cup ricotta cheese*
½ cup fat-free milk	*½ cup iceberg lettuce*		*½ cup tomato sauce with tomato bits*
1 cup orange juice	*2 slices tomato*		*1 ounce part-skim moz-zarella cheese*
	1 ounce low-fat cheddar cheese		1 ounce whole wheat dinner roll
	2 tbsp salsa		1 cup fat-free milk
	½ cup avocado		
	1 tsp lime juice		
	1 unsweetened beverage		

Breakfast	Lunch	Snacks	Dinner
(Choose one below)	*(Choose one below)*	*(Choose one below)*	*(Choose one below)*
1 whole wheat English muffin	Tuna fish sandwich	1 cup fat-free milk	Roasted chicken breast
2 tsp soft margarine	*2 slices rye bread*		*3 ounces boneless skinless chicken breast*
1 tbsp jam or preserves	*3 ounces tuna (packed in water, drained)*		1 large baked sweet potato
1 medium grapefruit	*2 tsp mayonnaise*		½ cup peas and onions
1 hard-cooked egg	*1 tbsp diced celery*		*1 tsp soft margarine*
1 unsweetened beverage	*¼ cup shredded romaine lettuce*		1 ounce whole wheat dinner roll
	2 slices tomato		*1 tsp soft margarine*
	1 medium pear		1 cup leafy greens salad
			3 tsp sunflower oil and vinegar dressing

Based on mypyramid.gov

Sample Weekly Menu Planner

Breakfast (about 300 calories)	Lunch (about 400 calories)	Dinner Choices (about 500 calories)	Snacks (about 150 calories)	Desserts (about 150 calories)
Choose one below	*Choose one below*	*Choose one below*	*Choose one below*	*Choose one below*

Breakfast (about 300 calories) — Choose one below

- Quick breakfast pizza
  Cooking spray
  1 egg plus 2 egg whites
  1 whole-grain pita (5 inches), toasted
  2 tbsp shredded part-skim mozzarella cheese
  ½ tsp dried oregano
  ½ cup grapes
  Make it: Spray skillet with cooking spray and scramble eggs. Top toasted pita with egg, cheese, and oregano. Broil for 5 minutes, until cheese is bubbling. Serve with grapes.

- Skillet pesto-potatoes and eggs
  Cooking spray
  ¾ cup finely chopped potatoes
  1 tbsp prepared pesto
  1 whole egg
  ½ medium grapefruit
  Make it: Spray skillet with cooking spray. Add potatoes and cook until golden, about 12 minutes, turning once. Toss potatoes with pesto and put on plate. Spray skillet with cooking spray again, cook egg, and place on top of potatoes. Serve with grapefruit.

- Breakfast burrito
  1 Amy's Breakfast Burrito (bought prepared)
  1 small peach
  Toast with walnut and pear spread
  ½ cup low-fat cottage cheese
  1 tbsp chopped walnuts
  ½ medium pear, finely chopped

Lunch (about 400 calories) — Choose one below

- Turkey, mozzarella, and basil wrap
  2 small (6-inch) whole-grain tortillas
  3 ounces turkey
  11-ounce slice part-skim mozzarella cheese, cut in half
  ¼ cup chopped fresh basil
  1 medium apple
  Make it: Fill tortillas with turkey, cheese, and basil. Serve with apple.

- White-bean gazpacho with whole-grain roll
  ½ cup canned white beans, rinsed and drained
  1 medium tomato, finely chopped
  1 cup finely chopped cucumber
  1 garlic clove, minced
  2 tbsp red-wine vinegar
  1 cup low-sodium tomato juice
  Dash of salt and pepper
  1 medium whole-grain roll
  Make it: Mix beans, tomato, cucumber, garlic, vinegar, tomato juice, and salt and pepper. Serve with roll.

- Asian tuna salad
  ¼ cup low-fat plain yogurt
  1 tsp wasabi powder
  ½ lime, juiced
  2 tsp olive oil
  1 tsp light soy sauce
  3 ounces tuna, packed in water
  2 cups napa cabbage, shredded
  ½ cup shredded carrots
  ¼ cup sliced almonds

Dinner Choices (about 500 calories) — Choose one below

- Cashew and coconut tofu stir-fry with brown rice
  1 tsp sesame oil
  1 1-inch slice ginger, minced
  1 garlic clove, minced
  2 ounces firm tofu, cubed
  1 cup frozen stir-fry vegetables
  ⅓ cup light coconut milk
  2 tbsp cashews, chopped
  ½ cup microwavable brown rice
  Make it: Heat oil, ginger and garlic in skillet for 1 minute. Add tofu and saute for 8 minutes, turning once or twice. Add vegetables, coconut milk, and cashews; cover and cook another 8 minutes. Microwave brown rice, then top with tofu and vegetable mixture.

- Parmesan pasta with asparagus and white beans
  2 ounces uncooked whole wheat pasta
  2 tsp olive oil
  2 garlic cloves, minced
  1½ cups bite-size pieces asparagus (about 10 spears)
  ¼ cup canned white beans, rinsed and drained
  4 tbsp grated Parmesan cheese
  Make it: Cook pasta. In a pan, saute oil, garlic, and asparagus for 4 minutes. Add beans and cook for 4 more minutes. Toss pasta with bean mixture and parmesan.

- Spinach-ricotta frittata with tossed green salad
  Cooking spray
  1½ cups baby spinach
  2 eggs plus 2 egg whites, whisked together

Snacks (about 150 calories) — Choose one below

- Spicy peanut spread on celery
  1 tbsp peanut butter
  Cayenne pepper to taste
  ½ lime, juiced
  4 medium celery stalks
  Make it: Mix peanut butter, cayenne, and lime juice. (To soften peanut butter, microwave it for 30 seconds.) Spread on celery.

- Honey-curry dip with carrots
  ⅓ cup low-fat plain yogurt
  1 tsp honey
  ½ tsp curry powder
  1 cup baby carrots
  Make it: Mix yogurt with honey and curry powder. Dip carrots.

- Corn chips and salsa verde
  10 corn chips
  2 tbsp prepared green salsa

- Yogurt with honey and sunflower seeds
  6 ounces low-fat plain yogurt
  1 tsp honey
  2 tsp sunflower seeds
  Make it: Mix all ingredients together.

- Mini ham and honey-mustard sandwiches
  1 tbsp honey-mustard salad dressing
  1 slice whole-grain bread, cut into 4 squares
  1 ounce low-fat ham
  Make it: Spread honey-mustard dressing on bread and top with ham. (Makes 2 mini sandwiches.)

- Grapefruit spritzer and soy nuts

Desserts (about 150 calories) — Choose one below

- Sauteed strawberry sundae
  1 tsp balsamic vinegar
  1 tsp honey
  ¼ cup sliced strawberries
  ½ cup light vanilla ice cream
  Make it: Saute vinegar, honey, and strawberries for 3 minutes. Top ice cream with warm berries.

- Grilled pineapple with gingersnap-crumb topping
  3 canned pineapple rings, packed in juice
  3 tbsp crushed gingersnap cookies (about 2 small cookies)
  Make it: Grill pineapple for 3 minutes on each side. Top with crushed cookies.

- Peach and blackberry crepe
  1 small peach, chopped
  ¼ cup low-fat cottage cheese
  1 premade crepe (found in the produce department)
  1 tbsp 100-percent blackberry fruit spread
  Make it: Mix together peaches and cottage cheese, then roll into crepe. Microwave fruit spread for 30 seconds and drizzle over crepe.

- Ice cream treat
  ½ cup Breyers Rocky Road Double Churn Light Ice Cream

  Dark-chocolate-covered graham crackers
  4 small graham-cracker rectangles
  2 tbsp semisweet chocolate chips

2 tsp honey
1 slice whole-grain bread, toasted
Make it: Mix cottage cheese, walnuts, pear, and honey (for smoother texture, puree in blender). Spread on toast.

- Waffle with fresh blueberries and lemon syrup

¾ cup blueberries
2 tsp maple syrup
½ lemon, juiced
1 whole-grain frozen waffle (4-inch), toasted
1 8-ounce glass skim or light soy milk
Make it: Mash blueberries with fork and mix with maple syrup and lemon juice. Top waffle with blueberry mixture. Serve with milk.

- Strawberry, banana, and flax smoothie

½ medium banana
½ cup frozen unsweetened strawberries
1 ½ cups skim milk or light soy milk
2 tbsp ground flaxseed
Make it: Blend all until smooth.

- Takeout!

From Au Bon Pain:
Medium oatmeal
Small fruit cup

Make it: Whisk together yogurt, wasabi, lime juice, olive oil, and soy sauce. Toss with tuna, cabbage, carrots, and almonds.

- Feta, hummus, and cucumber sandwich

⅔ cup canned chickpeas, rinsed and drained
½ lemon, juiced
1 garlic clove, minced
2 tbsp feta cheese
2 slices whole-grain bread
6 cucumber slices
Make it: With potato masher, mash chickpeas, lemon, garlic, and feta. Spread on bread and top with cucumber.

- Bruschetta burger with spinach salad

1 vegetarian burger
2 tbsp premade bruschetta spread
1 whole-grain hamburger bun
2 cups baby spinach
2 tbsp vinaigrette
Make it: Heat burger in microwave. Place on bun and top with bruschetta. Serve with spinach tossed with vinaigrette.

- Takeout!

From Taco Bell:
Fresco Ranchero Chicken Soft Taco
Fresco Grilled Steak Soft Taco
Side of guacamole

⅓ cup part-skim ricotta cheese
Dash of salt and pepper
2 cups romaine lettuce
2 tbsp pine nuts
2 tbsp low-fat Italian dressing
Make it: Spray skillet with cooking spray and saute spinach for 2 minutes, until wilted. Stir in eggs, ricotta, and salt and pepper. Cook over medium heat without stirring for 4 minutes; then flip frittata and cook for an additional 2 minutes. Serve with lettuce tossed with pine nuts and dressing.

- Curried quinoa salad with grilled shrimp

3 ounces frozen uncooked shrimp, thawed under running water for 5 minutes
1 tsp olive oil
¾ cup water
½ cup quinoa
¼ tsp curry powder
1 tbsp dried cranberries
1 cup chopped cucumbers
2 scallions, chopped
Make it: Toss shrimp with oil. Grill for 6 to 8 minutes, flipping once. Bring water and quinoa to a boil, cover, and simmer for 15 minutes. Stir in curry, cranberries, cucumbers, and scallions. Top with shrimp.

- Takeout!

From Chili's:
Guiltless Chicken Sandwich Meal (with black beans and steamed seasonal veggies)
From Ruby Tuesday:
Petite Sirloin
Creamy Mashed Cauliflower
Fresh Tomato and Mozzarella Salad

4 ounces 100-percent grapefruit juice
8 ounces sparkling water
¼ cup soy nuts
Make it: Stir together grapefruit juice and sparkling water. Serve with soy nuts.

- Crackers and goat cheese

6 whole-grain crackers
½ ounce goat cheese

Make it: Microwave chocolate chips for 30 seconds, until just melted. Spread graham crackers with chocolate and let sit for 10 minutes, until chocolate has hardened.

- Homemade mango-lime sorbet

½ cup frozen mango pieces
2 limes, juiced
1 tbsp honey
Make it: Puree ingredients in a blender until smooth and thick.

- Takeout!

From Starbucks:
Petite Vanilla Bean Scone
Grande Iced Coffee (unsweetened)

Guilt-Free Treats

- 2 Skinny Cow Vanilla and Caramel Skinny Dippers = 160 calories
- 1 VitaBrownie = 100 calories
- 2 Oatmeal Chocolate Chip Cookies (1 pack South Beach Living) = 100 calories
- ¾ cup Ciao Bella Raspberry Sorbetto = 150 calories
- 3 Firecracker Popsicles = 105 calories
- Weight Watchers English Toffee Crunch bar = 110 calories
- 1 Kraft Handi-Snacks Chocolate Pudding = 100 calories
- 1 Nabisco 100 Calorie Packs Mister Salty Milk Chocolate Covered Pretzels = 100 calories

ASSIGNMENT #10

Name: _____

Date: _____

1. Plan a weekly menu for yourself based on your *caloric needs*. Use additional pages if necessary.

Monday	Tuesday	Wednesday	Thursday	Friday

2. How can you help educate friends and family members to understand the components of a healthful diet?

_____

_____

_____

_____

_____

_____

_____

_____

_____

_____

_____

_____

_____

_____

_____

_____

_____

_____

3. How can you influence the food choices available in your school cafeteria?

_____

_____

_____

_____

_____

_____

_____

_____

_____

_____

_____

_____

_____

_____

_____

_____

RESOURCES

Agricultural Research Magazine, "Nutrition Research: Key To Eating Better" December 1999.

American Heart Association: www.americanheart.org.

Bouchard, C. (1997). Genetics of Human Obesity: Recent Results from Linkage Studies. *The Journal of Nutrition* 127, (9): 1887S–1890S.

Bray, G. (2002). Predicting Obesity in Adults from Childhood and Adolescent Weight. *The American Journal of Clinical Nutrition.* 76, (3): 497–498.

Byers, T., Nestle, M., McTiernan, A. et al. (2002). American Cancer Society guidelines on nutrition and physical activity for cancer prevention: reducing the risk of cancer with healthy food choices and physical activity. *CA: A Cancer Journal for Clinicians.* 52: 92–119.

Calle, E. E., Rodriguez, C., Walker-Thurmond, K.,Thun, M. J., (2003). Overweight, obesity and mortality from cancer in a prospectively studied cohort of U.S. adults. *New England Journal of Medicine.* 348(17):1625–1638.

Center for Science in the Public Interest: http://www.cspinet.org/.

Dansinger, M. L., Gleason, A. J., Griffith, J., Selker, H. P., Schaefer, E. J. (2005). Comparison of the Atkins, Ornish, Weight Watchers, and Zone Diets for Weight Loss and Heart Disease Risk Reduction. *Journal of the American Medical Association.* 293:43–53.

Duke University Diet and Fitness Center: www.dukedietcenter.org.

Fitness magazine, August 2008.

Glanz, K., Basil, M., Maibach, E., et al. (1998). Why Americans eat what they do: taste, nutrition, cost, convenience, and weight control concerns as influences on food consumption. *Journal of the American Dietetic Association.* 98:1118–26.

International Agency for Research on Cancer: http://www.iarc.fr/.

Jetter, K. M., Cassady, D. L.(2005). The availability and cost of healthier food alternatives. *American Journal of Preventive Medicine.* 30:38–44.

Mitchell, D. C., Shannon, B. M., McKenzie, J., et al. (2005). Lower fat diets for children did not increase food costs. *Journal of Nutrition Education.* 32:100–3.

National Heart Lung and Blood Institute: http://www.nhlbi.nih.gov/health/public/heart/obesity/lose_wt/shop_lst.htm.

Nutrition Analysis Tools and System: http://nat.crgq.com.

Portion Distortion slide sets: http://hp2010.nhlbihin.net/portion/.

Raynor, H. A., Kilanowski, C. K., Esterlis, I, Epstein, L. H. (2002). A cost-analysis of adopting a healthful diet in a family-based obesity treatment program. *Journal of the American Dietetic Association.* 102:645–50.

Spiegel, K., Tasali, E., Penev,P., Van Cauter, E. (2004). Sleep Curtailment in Healthy Young Men Is Associated with Decreased Leptin Levels, Elevated Ghrelin Levels, and Increased Hunger and Appetite. *Annals of Internal Medicine.* 141: 846–850.

Stroke Association: www.StrokeAssociation.org.

USDA Nutrient Data Laboratory: www.nal.usda.gov.

World Health Organization. (2000). Obesity: preventing and managing the global epidemic. Geneva: WHO.

World Health Organization Technical Report Series 916. (2003). Diet, nutrition and the prevention of chronic diseases: report of a joint FAO/WHO Expert Committee. Geneva: World Health Organization: http://whqlibdoc.who.int/trs/WHO_TRS_916.pdf.

HEALTHY RECIPES

11

Tuna-Stuffed Red Pepper Salad

Ingredients:

1 medium sweet red bell pepper

1 3-ounce can chunk light tuna in water, drained and flaked

1 small green onion, sliced (reserve a few slices for garnish, if desired)

¼ cup cooked brown rice

1 tbsp chopped celery or water chestnuts

2 tsp low-sodium soy sauce

½ tsp fresh grated ginger

2 tsp rice vinegar

½ tsp sesame oil

Salt, to taste

Directions:

Remove stem from red bell pepper and slice in half, lengthwise. Set aside half for another use. In a small bowl, mix together the tuna, green onion, cooked brown rice and celery or water chestnuts. Add the remaining ingredients and combine. Spoon tuna mixture into the pepper shell and garnish with reserved green onion slices. Serve slices of the red pepper with the tuna filling.

Nutrition Analysis per Serving:

Calories 228

Total Fat 4g

Sat. Fat 0.5g

Mono Fat 1g

Trans Fat 0g

Poly Fat 1.5g

Carbs 21g

Dietary Fiber 4g

Protein 25g

Sugars 5.5g

Sodium 758mg

Cholesterol 25.5mg

Vegetarian Stuffed Peppers

Ingredients:

4 green bell peppers

4 servings brown rice

1 can kidney or any type of bean (low sodium)

Boca or Morningstar vegetable ground crumbles

Salsa or diced tomatoes

Directions:

Core and clean peppers; place in microwave-safe dish with a little water in the bottom until they get somewhat soft. Make brown rice; add kidney or any type of bean and vegetable ground crumbles. Add any seasoning depending on desired spiciness and some salsa or diced tomatoes. Stuff mixture into peppers and bake for about 45 minutes or until lightly browned on top.

Nutrition Analysis per Serving:

Calories 350

Protein 24g

Carbs 58g

Total Fat 1.5g

Sodium 630mg

Fiber 12g

Chowder

Ingredients:

1 tbsp vegetable oil

1 cup onion, chopped

1 celery stalk, chopped

1 carrot, chopped

⅛ tsp cayenne pepper

½ tsp cumin

1 garlic clove, minced

2 cups fresh corn kernels (approximately 4 ears)

2 large, fresh tomatoes, chopped

1 small zucchini, quartered and sliced

1 ½ cup water

1 tsp salt

2 cup fresh spinach, chopped

1 ½ cup milk (1%)

2 tbsp fresh cilantro, minced

Directions:

Heat oil in a heavy 2-quart saucepan; sauté onion, celery, carrots, cayenne, cumin, and garlic until tender (5 to 7 minutes). Add corn, tomatoes, zucchini, water, and salt to sautéed vegetables. Bring to a boil; reduce heat to low. Cover and simmer for about 30 minutes until corn is tender. Add spinach, milk, and cilantro. Heat 5 minutes more over low heat. Thin with additional milk if necessary.

Nutrition Analysis per Serving:

Calories 189.81

Protein 7.75g

Carbs 30.98g

Total Fat 5.79g

Saturated Fat 1.29g

Cholesterol 5.63mg

Sodium 713.04mg

Fiber 4.79g

Asian Lettuce Wraps

Ingredients:

½ cup reduced-fat peanut butter

¼ cup honey

2 tbsp Hoisin sauce

2 tbsp water

2 tsp fresh lime juice

⅛ tsp ground red pepper

Cooking spray

1 lb skinless, boneless chicken breast halves

12 romaine lettuce leaves

2 cups julienne-cut carrots

1 cup julienne-cut seeded peeled cucumbers

1 cup fresh sprouts

Directions:

Combine first six ingredients in a bowl and whisk. Set aside. Coat a large, nonstick skillet with cooking spray and place over medium-high heat. Add chicken; thoroughly cook each side until done, cool, then slice into strips. Divide chicken evenly among lettuce leaves; top with carrot, cucumber, and sprouts. Roll up and serve with sauce.

Makes 6 servings (serving size: 2 wraps and 2 tbsp sauce)

Nutrition Analysis per Serving:

Calories 295.61

Protein 24.21g

Carbs 31.87g

Total Fat 9.28g

Saturated Fat 1.96g

Cholesterol 43.85mg

Sodium 369.13mg

Fiber 3.94g

Sautéed Spanish Chorizo

Ingredients:

6 to 8 oz roasted red pepper

4 oz chorizo

3 oz goat cheese

5 to 6 fresh basil leaves

1 clove fresh garlic, finely diced

2 tbsp white wine

Directions:

Roast peppers over an open flame until well charred, then place in a bowl and cover with plastic wrap. When the peppers are cool enough to handle, peel, seed, and julienne them. Dice chorizo into ¼-inch pieces. Heat about 1 ounce olive oil and begin to sauté the chorizo, draining any excess fat. Add roasted peppers, garlic, and white wine, finish with roughly chopped basil, and place into dish. Sprinkle with goat cheese and garnish with basil on top.

Nutrition Analysis per Serving:

Calories 228.77

Protein 11.49g

Carbs 4.53g

Total Fat 17.2g

Saturated Fat 8.47g

Cholesterol 41.74mg

Sodium 685.14mg

Fiber 0.04g

Turkey Wrap

Ingredients:

2 oz honey turkey

3 thin slices red onion

4 thin apple slices

2 slices cheddar cheese

1 tbsp garlic mayo (1 cup mayonnaise with 1 clove minced garlic)

1 red pepper tortilla

Makes 2 servings

Nutrition Analysis per Serving:

Calories 200

Protein 12g

Carbohydrates 9g

Total Fat 13g

Saturated Fat 4g

Cholesterol 50mg

Sodium 711mg

Fiber 5g

Chocolate Custard Cake

Ingredients:

Cake:

> Vegetable oil spray
>
> 14-oz can nonfat sweetened condensed milk
>
> Egg substitute equivalent to 5 eggs
>
> ½ cup 1% milk
>
> ½ cup Splenda
>
> ¼ cup nonfat or low-fat chocolate syrup

Topping:

> 1 ¼ cup seedless all-fruit preserves (fruit of choice)
>
> 10 oz fresh or frozen blueberries, thawed
>
> 1 tbsp powdered sugar (optional)

Directions:

Preheat the oven to 350° F. Spray an 8-inch nonstick round cake pan with vegetable oil spray. Cut a circle of parchment paper or wax paper to fit the bottom of the pan. Place paper in pan. If using wax paper, spray the top with vegetable oil spray.

In a large bowl, whisk together all cake ingredients. Pour into prepared pan.

Place the pan in the middle of a 12- × 17- × 1-inch jellyroll pan and fill jellyroll pan half full with warm water, or place cake pan in a baking pan (the bottom of a broiler pan works well), and add warm water to a depth of 1 inch.

Bake for 40 to 45 minutes, or until a toothpick inserted in the center of the cake comes out clean. Remove cake pan from water and let cool on a wire rack for 10 minutes. Carefully invert onto a plate (it is not necessary to loosen sides first) and remove paper.

Let cool for 15 minutes. While cake is cooling, heat preserves in a small saucepan over low heat, stirring occasionally.

Top the cake with a thin coating of the preserves. Sprinkle with about half of the blueberries. Cut the cake into 10 pie-shaped slices. Spoon remaining preserves on each dessert plate. Place each cake slice on preserves. Top with remaining blueberries, then dust lightly with powdered sugar.

For a more formal presentation, place blueberries in a ring around the top of the cake before cutting. Sprinkle any remaining berries on the dessert plates.

Makes 12 servings

Nutrition Analysis per Serving:

> Calories 269.13
>
> Protein 6.15g
>
> Carbs 60.87g
>
> Total Fat 0.28g
>
> Saturated Fat 0.14g
>
> Cholesterol 3.98m
>
> Sodium 115.19mg
>
> Fiber 0.82g

Vegetable Stew

Ingredients:

2 tbsp water

1 cup zucchini, thinly sliced

1-¼ cups yellow squash, thinly sliced

½ cup green bell pepper, cut into 2 inch strips

¼ cup celery, cut into 2 inch strips

¼ cup onion, chopped

½ tsp caraway seeds

⅛ tsp garlic powder

1 medium tomato, cut into 8 wedges

Directions:

Add first six ingredients to a heavy, nonstick skillet over medium heat. Cover and cook 4 minutes, or until vegetables are just tender. Add remaining ingredients, reduce heat to low, cover, and cook another 2 minutes.

Nutrition Analysis per Serving:

Calories 38

Fat 0.7g

Cholesterol 0mg

Protein 1.6g

Carbohydrates 8.6g

Fiber 2.6g

Sugar 4.6g

Sodium 13mg

Honey Dijon Spinach Salad

Ingredients:

1 lb. spinach leaves, washed and torn into pieces, tough stems discarded

2 cups mushrooms, sliced

1 cup cherry tomatoes, cut in half

¼ cup fat-free honey dijon dressing

Directions:

Combine spinach, mushrooms and tomatoes in a salad bowl. Pour dressing over salad and toss.

Nutrition Analysis per Serving:

Calories 67

Fat 0.7g

Cholesterol 0mg

Protein 4.6g

Carbohydrates 13.4g

Fiber 4.5g

Sugar 5.2g

Sodium 245mg

Baked Beans

Ingredients:

2 bacon slices (or turkey bacon) cut into 1-inch pieces (optional)

1-¼ lbs canned baked beans

⅓ cup onion, chopped

2 tbsp plus 2 tsp brown sugar, firmly packed

2 tsp molasses

1-¼ tsp Worcestershire sauce

¼ tsp dry mustard

Directions:

Heat a heavy, nonstick skillet over medium high heat. Sauté bacon 5 to 7 minutes, stirring frequently until crisp. Drain and discard drippings. Stir in remaining ingredients. Cover, reduce heat to medium low and **simmer** 15 minutes.

Nutrition Analysis per Serving:

Calories 183

Fat 0.7g

Cholesterol 0mg

Protein 7g

Carbohydrates 41.8g

Fiber 7.3g

Sugar 20.3g

Sodium 585mg

Sweet Whipped Potatoes

Ingredients:

¾ lb sweet potatoes, peeled and cut into 1 inch pieces

½ lb baking potatoes, peeled and cut into 1 inch pieces

¼ cup cottage cheese

¼ cup evaporated skim milk

¼ tsp salt (optional), or to taste

⅛ tsp pepper

Directions:

Place potatoes in steamer basket over boiling water. Cover and **steam** about 15 minutes or until tender. Remove potatoes from pan. Transfer to a mixing bowl. While potatoes are cooking, place cottage cheese in a food processor or blender and process until smooth. Transfer cottage cheese and remaining ingredients to potatoes. Beat with an electric mixer at medium speed until mixture is smooth.

Nutrition Analysis per Serving:

Calories 178

Fat 1.0g

Cholesterol 3mg

Protein 5.7g

Carbohydrates 37.2g

Fiber 3.7g

Sugar 8.0g

Sodium 91mg

Potato Salad

Ingredients:

1-¾ lbs small new potatoes

1 large egg, hard-cooked, peeled and chopped

3 tbsp fat-free mayonnaise

3 tbsp nonfat sour cream

¼ cup dill relish

1 tbsp scallions, finely chopped

2 tbsp prepared mustard

1 tsp dried tarragon

Directions:

Place potatoes in a steamer basket over boiling water. Cover pan and **steam** about 20 minutes or until just tender. Drain potatoes and rinse under cold running water to cool. Combine remaining ingredients with salt and pepper to taste in a bowl. Peel potatoes and cut into ½ inch dice and gently toss with egg mixture. Serve potato salad chilled or at room temperature.

This recipe serves 8 people. Due to the nature of this recipe, it adjusts the number of servings in multiples of 8 only.

Nutrition Analysis per Serving:

Calories 123

Fat 1.2g

Cholesterol 36mg

Protein 3.5g

Carbohydrates 25g

Fiber 2.0g

Sugar 4.2g

Sodium 170mg

Chicken Teriyaki

Ingredients:

2 chicken breasts, whole, split in half

½ cup soy sauce

¼ cup dry sherry

1 tbsp sugar

1 clove garlic, chopped

½ tsp ground ginger

Directions:

Arrange chicken, skin side up, in a single layer in a shallow dish. Combine soy sauce, sherry, sugar, garlic, and ginger in a jar with a tight-fitting lid. Shake vigorously and pour over chicken. Marinate in refrigerator 2 hours, turning once or twice. Preheat broiler. Remove chicken from marinade. Spray rack in broiler pan with vegetable spray. Transfer chicken to rack. Broil about 10 minutes about 6 inches from heat, turning once and basting with marinade.

Nutrition Analysis per Serving:

Calories 141

Fat 1.4g

Cholesterol 53mg

Protein 22.9g

Carbohydrates 6.5g

Fiber 0.3g

Sugar 4.6g

Sodium 1889mg

Japanese Soba Noodle Salad

Ingredients:

11 ounces soba noodles

2 scallions, minced

1 tbsp. plus 1 tsp fresh parsley, chopped

2 tsp mirin wine

2 tbsp lemon juice

¾ tsp fresh ginger, grated

¾ tsp garlic, pressed

1 tbsp plus 1 tsp yellow or white miso paste

1-¼ tsp sesame seeds

Directions:

Cook soba noodles in a large pan of boiling water about 5 minutes. Drain and rinse with cold water. Combine noodles, scallions and parsley in a bowl. Combine next 4 ingredients in a separate bowl. Then mix in miso, working out the lumps with the back of a spoon. Thin if necessary with a little water, drop by drop. Combine with noodle mixture and chill. Garnish with sesame seeds.

Nutrition Analysis per Serving:

Calories 110

Fat 1.1g

Cholesterol 0mg

Protein 5.4

Carbohydrates 21.0g

Fiber 2.0g

Sugar 1.3g

Sodium 259mg

Orange-Grilled Chicken with Herbs

Ingredients:

   2 cloves garlic, crushed

   ¾ tsp orange peel, grated

   ¼ tsp fresh thyme, minced

   ¼ tsp fresh rosemary, minced

   Freshly ground black pepper

   1 lb boneless chicken breast fillets, skin attached

   ⅓ cup fresh orange juice

   1 tbsp plus 1 tsp vinegar

   2 tsp Worcestershire sauce

Directions:

Combine the first 5 ingredients in a small bowl to make the herb mixture. Take each chicken breast and slip your fingers between the skin and flesh of the chicken, leaving the skin attached. Slide some of the herb mixture under the skin of each breast, pulling the skin back over each breast when finished. Prepare an outside grill with an oiled rack set 4 inches above the heat source.

   On a grill, set the heat to high. Mix together the orange juice, vinegar, and Worcestershire sauce in a small bowl. Grill the chicken breasts for 3–4 minutes on each side, turning once and basting with the orange juice mixture, until the chicken is cooked through. Remove the skin before eating.

Nutrition Analysis per Serving:

   Calories 140

   Fat 1.5g

   Cholesterol 66mg

   Protein 26.5g

   Carbohydrates 3.6g

   Fiber 0.1g

   Sugar 2.4g

   Sodium 102mg

Pasta Salad

Ingredients:

   2 cups cooked corkscrew macaroni

   1-⅓ cups chopped tomatoes

   ⅔ cup canned sweet corn kernels

   ⅔ cup canned black beans or red kidney beans, drained and rinsed

   ⅓ cup red onions, or purple onions

   3-½ tbsp chopped red bell pepper

   3-½ tbsp chopped green bell pepper

   3-½ tbsp chopped yellow bell pepper

   1-¼ tsp vinegar

¾ tsp lemon juice

¾ tsp olive oil

¾ tsp Italian herb seasoning

1 tbsp plus 1 tsp grated Parmesan or Romano cheese

⅛ tsp orange zest, optional

⅛ tsp salt (optional)

⅛ tsp black pepper (optional)

Directions:

Mix all ingredients in a large bowl. Keep refrigerated until served (up to 24 hours).

Nutrition Analysis per Serving:

Calories 173

Fat 2.3g

Cholesterol 1mg

Protein 7.2g

Carbohydrates 32.5g

Fiber 5.5g

Sugar 6.3g

Sodium 132mg

Shrimp Salad

Ingredients:

1 lb cooked shrimp, thawed and drained

1 cucumber, peeled, seeded and thinly sliced

12 radishes, thinly sliced

4 scallions, sliced

½ cup white wine vinegar

1 tbsp sugar

Directions:

Combine all ingredients in a bowl and toss well. Chill.

Nutrition Analysis per Serving:

Calories 181

Fat 2.6g

Cholesterol 196mg

Protein 27.7g

Carbohydrates 11.4g

Fiber 2.1g

Sugar 8.0g

Sodium 200mg

Grilled Pork Tenderloin

Ingredients:

4 pork tenderloin chops

½ tsp coarsely ground black pepper

⅔ cup orange marmalade

¼ cup fresh mint, chopped

¼ cup lite soy sauce

4 cloves garlic, crushed

Directions:

Prepare grill or turn on broiler. Butterfly tenderloin by cutting a lengthwise slit two-thirds of the way into each tenderloin, without cutting all the way through. Place tenderloin between 2 sheets of plastic wrap. Flatten slightly with a mallet or other heavy flat object. Sprinkle with pepper. Combine remaining ingredients in a small nonreactive saucepan. Brush mixture over tenderloin. Set aside remaining marmalade mixture. Grill or broil tenderloin about 8 minutes per side, basting frequently with marmalade mixture. Heat remaining marmalade mixture over medium heat about 1 minute, stirring until warm. Serve tenderloin with marmalade mixture.

Nutrition Analysis per Serving:

Calories 220

Fat 2.3g

Cholesterol 35mg

Protein 13.9g

Carbohydrates 38.3g

Fiber 0.4g

Sugar 34.9g

Sodium 589mg

Lower Fat Biscuits

Ingredients:

1-⅓ cups reduced fat buttermilk baking mix

½ cup skim milk

Directions:

Preheat oven to 450° F. Combine both ingredients in a bowl and stir until a soft dough forms. If dough is too sticky, gradually stir in enough baking mix (up to 1 tbsp plus 1 tsp) to make dough easy to handle. For rolled biscuits: Turn dough onto surface dusted with baking mix. Roll in baking mix to coat. Knead 10 times. Roll to ½ inch thick. Cut with a 2-½ inch cutter. Place on an ungreased cookie sheet. For drop biscuits: Do not knead dough. Drop by spoonfuls onto an ungreased cookie sheet. Bake 7 to 9 minutes or until golden brown.

Nutrition Analysis per Serving:

Calories 162

Fat 2.6g

Cholesterol 1mg

Protein 4.1g

Carbohydrates 29.8

Fiber 0.5g

Sugar 3.5g

Sodium 480mg

Sweet and Sour Chicken

Ingredients:

3 tbsp cornstarch

1-⅔ cups canned Asian or chicken stock

¼ cup vinegar

¼ cup sugar

1 lb boneless skinless chicken breast halves, cut into cubes

1 small green or red bell pepper, cut into 2-inch strips

1 medium carrots, sliced

½ lb unsweetened pineapple chunks, drained

4 cups hot cooked rice

Directions:

Combine first 4 ingredients in a bowl until smooth. Set aside. Heat a heavy nonstick skillet over medium high heat. Stir-fry chicken 5 to 8 minutes, in batches if necessary, or until browned. Set chicken aside.

Stir cornstarch mixture and add to skillet. Cook until mixture boils and thickens, stirring constantly. Return chicken to pan. Add pepper, carrot and pineapple. Reduce heat to low. Cover and cook 5 minutes or until chicken is no longer pink. Serve over rice.

This recipe serves 4 people. Due to the nature of this recipe, it adjusts the number of servings in multiples of 4 only.

Nutrition Analysis per Serving:

Calories 494

Fat 2.8g

Cholesterol 66mg

Protein 33.8g

Carbohydrates 81.2g

Fiber 2.2g

Sugar 21.4g

Sodium 412mg

Grilled Chicken Kabobs

Ingredients:

¼ cup water

2 tbsp soy sauce

2 tbsp. lemon juice

1 tbsp honey

¼ tsp garlic powder

¼ tsp ground ginger

4 boneless skinless chicken breast halves, cut into 1-½ inch pieces skewers

1 green bell pepper, seeded and cut into 1-½ inch pieces

1 onion, quartered

8 large cherry tomatoes

Directions:

Combine first 6 ingredients in a glass baking dish. Add chicken and turn to coat. Cover and marinate at least 2 hours in refrigerator. Prepare grill. Remove chicken from marinade and boil marinade 10 minutes in a saucepan. Alternate chicken and vegetables on skewers. Grill 6 inches from medium-hot coals 15 to 20 minutes, or until done, turning and basting often with marinade.

Nutrition Analysis per Serving:

Calories 323

Fat 3.7g

Cholesterol 106mg

Protein 46.4g

Carbohydrates 28.2g

Fiber 5.0g

Sugar 18.1g

Sodium 611mg

Broccoli with Breadcrumbs

Ingredients:

1 lb broccoli florets

2 tsp unsalted butter

½ cup seasoned breadcrumbs

2 tbsp parsley, finely chopped

Directions:

Place broccoli in a steamer basket over boiling water. Cover saucepan and steam 5 to 6 minutes or until bright green and tender.

Drain and transfer to a serving dish. Keep warm. Melt butter in a heavy nonstick skillet over medium heat. Add breadcrumbs and stir until butter is absorbed. Sprinkle broccoli with breadcrumbs and parsley. Toss lightly.

Nutrition Analysis per Serving:

Calories 104

Fat 2.7g

Cholesterol 5mg

Protein 5.6g

Carbohydrates 16.4g

Fiber 4.0g

Sugar 2.5g

Sodium 428mg

Chicken Marsala

Ingredients:

1-¼ tsp olive oil

¾ medium onion, chopped

1 lb boneless skinless chicken breast halves, pounded to ¼ inch thickness

⅔ cup dry Marsala wine

½ cup chicken stock, low-fat, low-sodium

2 tsp cornstarch, or arrowroot powder

salt and pepper

Directions:

In a large skillet over medium-high heat, heat the oil. Add the onion and sauté for 5 minutes. Add the chicken and cook on each side for 5 minutes. Add the wine and cook for about 4 minutes until the wine looks syrupy. In a small cup, dissolve the cornstarch or arrowroot powder in the stock. Add to the chicken and cook until the sauce is thickened, about 2 minutes. Add salt and pepper to taste.

Nutrition Analysis per Serving:

Calories 187

Fat 3.0g

Cholesterol 66mg

Protein 27.3g

Carbohydrates 4.8g

Fiber 0.4g

Sugar 2.3g

Sodium 175mg

Corn Muffins

Ingredients:

1 egg, lightly beaten

1 cup lowfat milk

½ tsp vanilla extract

2 tbsp vegetable oil

½ cup cornmeal

¾ cup flour

¼ cup sugar

1-½ tsp baking powder

½ tsp salt (optional)

Directions:

Preheat oven to 400° F. Combine egg, milk, vanilla, oil and cornmeal in a mixing bowl. Mix thoroughly. Let stand 10 minutes. Sift remaining ingredients together in another bowl. Add to cornmeal mixture. Mix thoroughly, without overworking. Fill greased muffin tins ⅔ full with batter. Bake 15 minutes, or until tester comes out clean when inserted in center of muffin. Cool 3 minutes in pan before turning muffins out. This recipe serves 12 people.

Nutrition Analysis per Serving:

Calories 96

Fat 3.1g

Cholesterol 16mg

Protein 2.3g

Carbohydrates 14.9g

Fiber 0.6g

Sugar 5.3g

Sodium 17mg

Low-Fat Coffee Cake

Ingredients:

⅓ cup brown sugar, packed

½ tsp ground cinnamon

1-¾ cups reduced-fat buttermilk baking mix

¾ cup skim milk

¼ cup sugar

1 tbsp unsalted butter, melted

1 egg

Directions:

Preheat oven to 375° F. Prepare streusel topping by combining first 2 ingredients in a bowl until crumbly. Set aside. Combine remaining ingredients in another bowl and stir until blended. Spread in a greased 9 inch round pan. Sprinkle with streusel topping. Bake 18 to 23 minutes or until golden brown.

Nutrition Analysis per Serving:

Calories 150

Fat 3.0g

Cholesterol 22mg

Protein 2.8g

Carbohydrates 28.0g

Fiber 0.3g

Sugar 14.2g

Sodium 262mg

Bean Soup

Ingredients:

1 tbsp Extra Virgin Olive Oil

1 medium Onion, coarsely chopped

1 medium carrot, peeled and diced

1 celery stalk, trimmed, diced

3 cloves garlic, chopped finely

3 cups vegetable broth

¼-cup ground flaxseed

15 ounce can cooked beans (Navy or Great Northern), washed and drained

Salt and pepper, to taste

Fresh chopped parsley, for garnish

Directions:

Preheat your stockpot, then add oil, onion, carrot, and celery. Over medium heat, sauté these vegetables for 5 to 8 minutes, until the pieces are lightly browned. Add the garlic, and continue to sauté for another minute.

Add the ground flaxseed and the vegetable broth, then simmer the whole mixture covered for about 15 minutes, being careful to keep the pot from reaching a boil. Add beans, salt and pepper (to taste), and continue cooking for about 5 minutes more. Ladle into serving bowls and garnish with fresh parsley. Accompany each bowl with a slice of whole grain bread for a satisfyingly filling meal.

Nutrition Analysis per Serving:

Calories 176

Fiber 8g

Carbohydrates 23g

Calcium 85mg

Protein 9g

Sodium 589mg

Fat 6g

Cholesterol: 0g

Veggie Quiche

Ingredients:

2 whole eggs

6 egg whites

¾ cup skim milk

1 oz low-fat cheddar cheese, shredded

1 ½ cup raw spinach

¾ cup raw, chopped green pepper

¾ cup raw, chopped onion

¾ cup raw, chopped zucchini squash

¾ cup tomato, diced

1 tbsp minced garlic

Dash of salt and pepper

Directions:

Preheat oven to 375° F. Cook spinach according to directions. Drain. Spray 9-inch pie pan with cooking spray to prevent sticking. Combine eggs and milk with a wire whisk in a large mixing bowl. Mix in the green pepper, onion, squash, tomatoes, garlic, salt, and pepper. Fold in the shredded cheddar cheese. Pour all ingredients into 9-inch pie pan. Bake at 375° F for 25 to 30 minutes until knife comes out clean.

Nutrition Analysis per Serving:

Calories 83

Protein 10g

Carbs 6g

Total Fat 2g

Saturated Fat 1g

Cholesterol 76mg

Sodium 167mg

Fiber 1g

Pumpkin Muffins

Ingredients:

1 ½ cup whole wheat flour

½ cup ground flax seed

2 tsp baking soda

1 tsp cloves

1 tsp cinnamon

½ tsp salt

1 cup chopped nuts

Optional: ½ cup semi-sweet chocolate chips

Directions:

Preheat oven to 350 degrees F and mix the dry ingredients together.

2 cups pumpkin

½ cup plain yogurt

¾ cup honey

1 tsp molasses

2 eggs

Beat the eggs and mix together with other wet ingredients. Mix the wet and dry ingredients together. Place in greased muffin tins. Bake for 20 to 25 minutes until dry to an inserted toothpick. Makes approximately 15 muffins.

Nutrition Analysis per Serving:

Calories 240

Carbohydrates 34g

Protein 6g

Dietary fiber 5g

Total fat 11g

Spanish Omelet

Ingredients:

5 small potatoes, peeled and sliced

1 tbsp olive oil or vegetable cooking spray

½ medium onion, minced

1 small zucchini, sliced

1-½ cup green/red peppers, sliced thin

5 medium mushrooms, sliced

3 whole eggs, beaten

5 egg whites, beaten

Pepper and garlic salt with herbs, to taste

3 ounces shredded part-skim mozzarella cheese

1 tbsp parmesan cheese

Directions:

Preheat oven to 375° F.

Cook potatoes in boiling water until tender. In a nonstick pan, add oil or vegetable spray and warm at medium heat. Add the onion and sauté until brown. Add vegetables and sauté until tender but not brown. In a medium mixing bowl, slightly beat the eggs and egg whites, pepper, garlic salt, and mozzarella cheese. Stir egg-cheese mixture into the cooked vegetables. Oil or spray a 10-inch pie pan or ovenproof skillet. Transfer potatoes and eggs mixture to pan. Spread with parmesan cheese and bake omelet until firm and brown on top, about 20–30 minutes.

Nutrition Analysis per Serving:

Calories 242

Carbohydrates 18g

Protein 19g

Fat 9g

Beef or Turkey Stew

Ingredients:

1 lb lean beef or turkey breast cut into cubes

Whole wheat flour

¼ tsp salt (optional)

¼ tsp pepper

¼ tsp cumin

1 ½ tbsp olive oil

2 cloves of garlic, minced

2 medium onions, sliced

2 stalks celery, sliced

1 medium red/green bell pepper, sliced

1 medium tomato, finely minced

5 cups of beef or turkey broth, fat removed

5 small potatoes, peeled and cubed

12 small carrots

1-¼ cups green peas

Directions:

Preheat oven to 375° F.

Mix the whole wheat flour with salt, pepper, and cumin, and roll the beef or turkey cubes in the mixture. Shake off excess flour. In a large skillet, heat the olive oil over medium-high heat. Add the beef or turkey cubes and sauté until nicely brown, about 7–10 minutes. Place the beef or turkey in an ovenproof casserole. Add minced garlic, onions, celery, and peppers to the skillet and cook until vegetables are tender, about 5 minutes.

Stir in the tomato and broth. Bring to a boil and pour over the turkey or beef pieces. Cover the casserole tightly and bake for 1 hour at 375° F. Remove from the oven and stir in the potatoes, carrots, and peas. Bake for another 20–25 minutes, or until tender.

Nutrition Analysis per Serving:

Calories 326

Carbohydrates 21g

Protein 27g

Fat 15g

Caribbean Red Snapper

Ingredients:

2 tbsp olive oil

1 medium onion, chopped

½ cup chopped red pepper

½ cup carrots, cut in strips

1 clove garlic, minced

½ cup dry white wine

¾ lb red snapper fillet

1 large tomato, chopped

2 tbsp pitted ripe olives, chopped

2 tbsp crumbled feta cheese or low-fat ricotta cheese

Directions:

In a large skillet, heat olive oil over medium heat. Add onion, red pepper, carrot, and garlic; sauté 10 minutes. Add wine and bring to boil. Push vegetables to one side of the pan. Arrange fillets in a single layer in center of skillet. Cover; cook for 5 minutes. Add tomato and olives. Top with cheese. Cover; cook 3 minutes, or until fish is firm but moist. Transfer fish to serving platter; garnish with vegetables and pan juices.

Nutrition Analysis per Serving:

Calories 193

Carbohydrates 3g

Protein 22g

Fat 11g

Two Cheese Pizza

Ingredients:

Whole wheat flour

1 can (10 oz) refrigerated pizza crust

2 tbsp olive oil

½ cup low-fat ricotta cheese

½ tsp dried basil

1 small onion, minced

2 cloves garlic, minced

¼ tsp salt (optional)

4 ounces shredded part-skim mozzarella cheese

2 cups chopped mushrooms

1 large red pepper, cut into strips

Directions:

Preheat oven to 425° F.

Spread whole-wheat flour over working surface. Roll out dough with rolling pin to desired crust thickness. Coat cookie sheet with cooking spray. Transfer pizza crust to cookie sheet. Brush olive oil over crust. Mix the ricotta cheese with the dried basil, onion, garlic, and salt; spread this mixture over crust. Sprinkle crust with mozzarella cheese. Top cheese with mushrooms and red pepper. Bake at 425° F for 13 to 15 minutes until cheese melts and crust is deep golden brown. Cut into 8 slices.

Nutrition Analysis per Serving:

Calories 351

Carbohydrates 34g

Protein 18g

Fat 16g

Eggplant Lasagna

Ingredients:

1 tbsp olive oil

1 medium onion, sliced

1 clove garlic, minced

1 large tomato, sliced very thin

1 cup canned crushed tomatoes

1 ½ tsp dried basil

1 ½ tsp dried oregano

¼ tsp salt (optional)

1 medium eggplant, sliced very thin

8 ounces shredded part-skim mozzarella cheese

Directions:

Preheat oven to 425° F.

In a medium nonstick skillet, heat olive oil over medium heat. Sauté onion until tender, about 2–3 minutes. Transfer to an 8×8 or 9×13 baking dish. Sauté the garlic for 1 minute. Add the crushed tomato, basil, oregano, and salt, and cook gently over medium-low heat for 10 minutes. Spread a layer of this mixture over the onion layer. Add a layer of eggplant and follow with a layer of tomato. Sprinkle ⅓ of the mozzarella cheese over top. Repeat layers of eggplant, tomato, and cheese until you use all ingredients. Finish with a layer of mozzarella cheese. Cover with aluminum foil and bake for 25 minutes, or until vegetables are tender. Uncover and bake 10 to 15 minutes, or until layer of cheese is light brown.

Nutrition Analysis per Serving:

Calories 219

Carbohydrates 5g

Protein 16g

Fat 15g

Rice with Chicken, Spanish Style

Ingredients:

2 tbsp olive oil

2 medium onions, chopped

4 garlic cloves, minced

2 stalks celery, diced

2 medium red/green peppers, cut into strips

1 cup chopped mushrooms

2 cups uncooked rice

1 3-lb chicken, cut into 8 pieces, skin removed

1 tsp salt (optional)

3 ½ cups chicken broth, fat removed

4 cups water Saffron or Sazón, for color

3 medium tomatoes, chopped

1 cup frozen peas

1 cup frozen corn

1 cup frozen green beans

Olives or capers for garnish, if desired

Directions:

Heat the oil over medium heat in a nonstick pot. Add the onion, garlic, celery, green pepper, and mushrooms. Cook over medium heat, stirring often, for about 3 minutes or until tender. Add the rice and sauté for 2 to 3 minutes, stirring constantly until it begins to brown. Add the chicken, salt, chicken broth, water, saffron (Sazón), and tomatoes. Bring the water to a boil, then reduce heat to medium-low and let simmer. Cover the pot and let the casserole simmer until the water is absorbed and rice is tender, about 20 minutes. Stir in the peas, corn, and beans, and cook for 8 to 10 minutes. When everything is hot the casserole is ready to serve. Garnish with olives or capers, if desired.

Nutrition Analysis per Serving:

Calories 330

Carbohydrates 24g

Protein 27g

Fat 14g

Seafood Stew

Ingredients:

6 cups water

10 oz white wine

3 celery stalks, chopped

3 medium carrots, chopped

1 lb large shrimp, washed

1 lb crayfish

2 tbsp olive oil

2 medium onions, chopped

1 medium red pepper, chopped

1 medium green bell pepper, chopped

4 medium tomatoes, chopped

2 tbsp tomato paste

2 tsp chopped fresh thyme

2 tsp chopped fresh oregano

1 lb sea bass, cut into chunks

1 lb small squid, cleaned and sliced

Salt and pepper to taste

Directions:

In a large, non-aluminum saucepan, stir together the water, white wine, celery, and carrots. Bring to a simmer and cook for 5 minutes. Add the shrimp and crayfish and simmer for 3 to 4 minutes. Strain the shellfish and vegetables from the broth and set the broth aside. Peel the crayfish and shrimp and discard the shells. Warm the olive oil in the large saucepan over medium-high heat. Cook the onions and peppers until tender, about 6 minutes. Stir in the tomatoes, tomato paste, thyme and oregano. Add the reserved broth and bring to a simmer. Stir in the sea bass and squid and simmer for 2 minutes. Return the crayfish, shrimp and vegetables to the broth and simmer for 1 more minute. Season to taste, ladle into bowls, and serve immediately.

Nutrition Analysis per Serving:

Calories 222

Carbohydrates 3g

Protein 36g

Fat 8g

Resources

American Diabetes Association's *Flavorful Seasons Cookbook: Great-Tasting Recipes for Winter, Spring, Summer and Fall* (1996) McGraw-Hill Companies.

Golden Valley Flax: www.flaxhealth.com.

National Institutes of Health: www.ndep.nih.gov.

Today's Diet and Nutrition: www.todaysdiet&nutrition.com.

INDEX